MUSCLE EXPLOSION

28 DAYS TO MAXIMUM MASS

The information found in this book does not constitute medical advice and should not be taken as such. Consult your physician before taking part in any exercise program. The dietary modifications found in this program are extreme and assume a healthy body. If you have medical considerations that require special nutritional practices, please review this book with your nutritionist and physician before starting.

Any application of the recommended material in this book is at the sole risk of the reader, and at the reader's discretion. Responsibility of any injuries or other adverse effects resulting from the application of any of the information provided within this book is expressly disclaimed.

PUBLISHED BY
Price World Publishing, LLC
1300 W. Belmont Ave, Suite 20G
Chicago, IL 60657

Modeling by   Nick Nilsson
Layout Design by   Raja Sekar
Photos by   Kelly Anderson
Book Cover by Dianne T Goh
Editing by   Lisa Reuter
Printing by   United Graphics, Inc.
Proofreading by   Rob Price

ISBN: 978-0-9724102-9-8
Library of Congress Control Number: 2010920935
First Edition, January 2011

Printed in the United States of America

10 9 8 7 6 5 4 3 2 1

MUSCLE EXPLOSION

28 DAYS TO MAXIMUM MASS

By Nick Nilsson

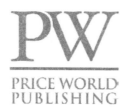

PRICE WORLD PUBLISHING

CONTENTS

Foreword

Michael Lipowski

If you are serious about building muscle, you know how difficult it is to move from the intermediate to advanced stages of training. Most people experience a training "honeymoon" period. During this time, you can add more weight to your lifts, increase the number of repetitions, or both, and know that muscle mass and strength gains follow. Like two old friends having a beer at a bar and reminiscing about high school, you could say that those were the "best of times."

Then reality sets in. You realize that making further progress will require much more work. It's at this point that most trainees make the fatal mistake of simply doing more of what's no longer working. The payoff for the increased time and effort in the gym is not new muscle, but frustration and a hopeless feeling that you've reached the limit of your genetic potential.

It's easy to fall into this situation. Heck, people continue down the same path in most areas of life without ever thinking about trying something new. Why would their behavior at the gym be any different? It's human nature.

We get used to doing things a certain way because it once worked, which makes it that much harder to change.

But as Nick Nilsson demonstrates throughout *Muscle Explosion: 28 Days to Maximum Mass*, breaking away from what you've acclimated to and "breaking the rules" is precisely what you *need to do* to reach the upper limits of muscle and strength development. Nilsson illustrates how achieving good results is not just a matter of doing things differently, as many other fitness professionals have suggested (and you may have already tried). It requires the systematic, scientific manner in which training and nutrition are *combined*. This makes Nick's program successful where others have failed.

Before I continue, let me be totally clear and brutally honest: I have never been a fan of predetermined training programs. The fact is that as individuals we vary greatly in our needs and abilities. So when I first opened Nick's book, I was skeptical about how effective this program could be for *anyone*, especially advanced trainees, wanting to add muscle mass and overcome strength plateaus. Nevertheless, as I began reading about the different training and nutrition strategies he employs and the science and rationale behind them, it became obvious that this program *can* work and *will* work for anyone who takes on the challenge. What I found most intriguing, as you probably will, is the way that Nick puts all the pieces of the muscle-building puzzle together for a predictable, desirable outcome.

If you asked me to name the most essential components for building muscle mass and strength, I would say without hesitation:

- Disrupting homeostasis (i.e., what your body has adapted to and considers normal).

- Striking a balance between exercise demands (stress) and recovery.

- A nutrition plan built around proper, precise macronutrients and meal timing.

- Tremendous mental focus.

- An extremely high intensity approach to training.

This program has it all!

While the approach seems unconventional at times, it does exactly what is most important to disrupting homeostasis. Sometimes it feels like you're doing too little or too much exercise. Yet that's just what is most important to balancing the demands (stress) of training with adequate recovery.

Nick's approach to nutrition seems unusual, but every step has a specific purpose to ensure you give your body exactly what it needs when it needs it. This will maximize the effectiveness of the training and amass quality muscle without accumulating body fat. While the training itself takes gut-busting effort and concentration, that's simply the price you must pay to experience real, *muscle-exploding results.*

Enjoy those results, and enjoy the journey.

Michael Lipowski, trainer of Men's Fitness magazine's first ever "Fat-to-Fit" contest winner, is a competitive natural bodybuilder and the president of the International Association of Resistance Trainers. His highly praised book, **Pure Physique: How to Maximize Fat-Loss and Muscular Development,** *can be found at bookstores nationwide. See the back of this book for information on how to get* **Pure Physique** *for 50% off.*

Introduction

This is a training manual about building muscle and strength EXPLOSIVELY FAST while minimizing fat gain.

It's about getting extremely fast, extremely powerful results by doing almost EVERYTHING WRONG, according to conventional wisdom!

Here it is up front: I'm NOT going to take up your time going into great detail about a bunch of things you probably already know about muscle building and training. I AM, however, going to go into great detail about how these groundbreaking training and eating strategies can SHATTER your "genetic limitations" by CHANGING YOUR PHYSIOLOGY and taking advantage of ALL the growth processes your body has available.

The Muscle Explosion Program is about BREAKING THE RULES and getting AMAZING results by doing so.

You'll use highly targeted, strategic changes in both training techniques AND nutrition to achieve these EXTREMELY RAPID RESULTS (adding 10 solid pounds in a month is not unrealistic), because if you want to grow FAST and KEEP growing like a weed, you need to constantly keep your body off balance.

But here's the kicker: You have to do it not only with change, you have to do it with INTELLIGENT change. Because let's face it, anyone can start mixing things around in their training without any regard for how one thing affects another. To get maximum results, you need to know how to build a foundation, then how to properly build ON that foundation.

To start, here are some of the things you're going to do "wrong"–or at least opposed to conventional muscle-building wisdom:

You're going to REDUCE your caloric intake to well below maintenance levels.

- You're going to eliminate protein from your diet (in a very specific way).

- You're going to do VERY high rep sets (30+ reps per set).

- You'll also do very LOW rep sets (three reps per set) with very little rest in between.

- You're going to train the same body part five days in a row.

- You're going to do the same EXERCISE five days in a row.

- You're going to learn how to train with heavy weight AND for high reps.

- You're going to stretch your muscles without doing any stretching.

- You're going to do a LOT of cardio, then you're going to do NONE.

- You're NOT going to stuff yourself full of food constantly, just strategically.

- You're going to stay away from muscular failure, then go FAR beyond it.

Put all these "wrong" things together in the RIGHT way and you're going to get EXPLOSIVE results.

How and Why I Developed this Program

It all started for me when I was 16 years old. I was a cross-country runner weighing in at a skinny 145 pounds. But that's not what I wanted to look like.

I wanted to be BIG and ripped like the guys I saw in the muscle magazines.

My quest to learn the best muscle-building techniques and information that would help me build massive muscle FAST would take me through five years of University education, graduating with a degree in Physical Education.

It would also take me through 10 years of my own personal research, constant reading and a willingness to push my body to the limit to discover the absolute best methods for maximizing muscle mass as quickly as humanly possible.

It was this non-stop research, this drive to be massive and strong and the willingness to use myself as a guinea pig that led me to develop the fundamentals of the Muscle Explosion training protocols you now hold in your hands.

I developed this program because I'm basically impatient.

I KNEW how to get muscle-building results over time; what I wanted was a program that would do it EXTREMELY fast, accomplishing results in just one month similar to what most programs only achieve in four to six months. It's a plateau-busting program that works for everyone, from the most advanced bodybuilder to the toughest hard-gainer.

And make no mistake; this program will push your body to the limits. It is not for beginners. It will show you what your body is truly capable of when you give it NO choice but to grow.

How to Use This Book

Start by reading through The Muscle Explosion Program. This section includes an overview of how the program works and how all the pieces fit together. It then includes the chart of workouts to follow. Subsequent sections provide more detailed information about exercise techniques and nutritional aspects of the program.

Be sure to read through all the sections before you start the program so you fully understand it and how it works. This will help you get the best results.

If you ever have any questions, please feel free to contact me at ANY time. I'm here to help, and nobody understands this program better than I do. My email address is betteru@fitstep. com.

Enjoy!

THE MUSCLE EXPLOSION PROGRAM

If you've been training awhile, you know that one of the biggest killers in any program is stagnation. As the old saying goes, "everything works but nothing works forever." This is where THIS program delivers the knockout punch!

This program uses the Macronutrient Rotation Principle as outlined in the Nutrition section, and the unique training techniques found in the Exercise section. They are powerful when taken separately. When you combine them to synergistically take advantage of the best of each, and add the power of proper transitioning between techniques, the results are tremendous. Note: I recommend you take at least four to seven full days off from any training before starting this program. You'll need it.

The Muscle Explosion Program consists of three phases, taking place over four weeks.

Phase 1

Week 1: Metabolic Acceleration and Tissue Remodeling Training

This week focuses on low-carb eating and training geared toward fat loss and depleting glycogen stores. Sounds strange for a muscle-building program to start with a strict fat-loss phase, doesn't it?

Here's the deal: We're going to use this low-calorie phase to set your body up for a big rebound. If you've ever been on a fat-loss diet, you know how much of a rebound you get when you switch back to higher-calorie eating. We're going to AMPLIFY the good parts of that rebound for the purposes of muscle growth.

This week's training is targeted not only for fat loss but to set up your body's physiology for optimal muscle growth in the next two phases.

Phase 2

Week 2: 5-Day Structural Attack

In this phase, you choose ONE exercise and one exercise ONLY. You're going to do LOTS of sets of it, and you're going to get VERY good and VERY strong with it. I HIGHLY recommend using squats or deadlifts the first time you go through this program. You'll get the most bang for your buck in terms of overall muscle growth using one of these two exercises. Nutritionally, you're going to come out of your low-calorie, fat-loss phase and start eating A LOT. Your body will be loading up on carbs, protein, and water (from creatine and glutamine loading). Your body will literally be SWIMMING in anabolic factors. Your body will be primed for maximum growth, and this training takes full advantage of it.

Phase 3

Weeks 3 and 4: Stretch-Pause Training

You'll continue the muscle-building effects of Phase 2, but instead of focusing on one exercise, you'll perform many different exercises. In these two weeks, you'll use a specialized training technique I call Stretch-Pause Training.

The name is a derivative of Rest-Pause Training. But instead of doing that exercise, you're going to use a stretch-accentuated attack on the target muscle, then move to a contraction-accentuated attack on that muscle. It's an INTENSE technique that will blow up your muscles like crazy!

After the Four Weeks Are Finished

If you have just finished your first round through the program, you can return to Week 1 and begin another 28-day cycle. For the second cycle, choose a different exercise for the 5-Day Structural Attack, for example, bench press, shoulder press, barbell rows, etc.

If you've just completed your second cycle, take a week completely OFF training. This is NOT optional. This program will seriously challenge your recovery ability. It attacks not only your muscles, but your connective tissue and nervous system. You will NEED the week off to fully recover. Don't worry. You won't lose your hard-won strength. In fact, you'll most likely INCREASE it further with the increased recovery.

Training Schedule

Everything for each training day is listed in a specific order. Follow the instructions as closely as possible to get the best results. The following charts show how the program is laid out.

Remember, read through the whole program first, so these charts make sense.

Muscle Explosion Weekly Training & Nutrition Charts

Phase 1

Week 1: Metabolic Acceleration and Tissue Remodeling Training

	DAY 1	DAY 2	DAY 3
WEIGHT TRAINING	Chest (3) sets Back (3) Thighs (3) Shoulders (2) Hamstrings (2) Biceps (2) Triceps (2) Calves (2) Fat Loss Circuit Training Style 40 seconds cardio Core Combo	Chest (4) Back (4) Thighs (4) Shoulders (3) Hamstrings (3) Biceps (3) Triceps (3) Calves (3) Fat Loss Circuit Training Style 20 seconds cardio Core Combo	No Weights
CARDIO TRAINING	No Cardio	No Cardio	No Cardio
NUTRITION	Low Carb	Low Carb	Low-Fat, High-Carb - But STILL LOW CALORIE

See the Appendix or visit www.sportsworkout. com/muscleexplosioncharts for daily training & nutrition charts.

	DAY 4	DAY 5
WEIGHT TRAINING	Chest (8 + 2) Back (8 + 2) Biceps (6 + 2) Calves (6 + 2) Traps (2) Lactic Acid Training Style	Shoulders (6 + 2) Triceps (6 + 2) Hamstrings (6 + 2) Thighs (8 + 2) Traps (2) Lactic Acid Training Style
CARDIO TRAINING	No Cardio	No Cardio
NUTRITION	Low Carb	Low Carb

	DAY 6	DAY 7
WEIGHT TRAINING	Core Combo	No Weights
CARDIO TRAINING	Interval Training	No Cardio
NUTRITION	Only Protein	Only Fruit

See the Appendix or visit www.sportsworkout. com/muscleexplosioncharts for daily training & nutrition charts.

Phase 2
Week 2 (Intermediate Program): 5-Day Structural Attack

This is the intermediate variation of this phase of the program. It consists of three training days with a day of rest between each training day.

	DAY 8	DAY 9
WEIGHT TRAINING	20 minutes of Compound Exercise; Overload on Target Exercise	No Weights
CARDIO TRAINING	No Cardio	No Cardio
NUTRITION	Moderate Fat, High Carb, High Protein	Moderate Fat, High Carb, High Protein

	DAY 11	DAY 12	DAY 13 AND 14
WEIGHT TRAINING	30 minutes of Compound Exercise; Overload on Target Exercise	No Weights	40 minutes of Compound Exercise; Overload on Target Exercise
CARDIO TRAINING	No Cardio		
NUTRITION	Moderate Fat, High Carb, High Protein	Moderate Fat, High Carb, High Protein	Moderate Fat, High Carb, High Protein

See the Appendix or visit www.sportsworkout. com/muscleexplosioncharts for daily training & nutrition charts.

Week 2 (Advanced Program): 5-Day Structural Attack

This is the advanced variation of this phase of the program. It consists of five training days in a row.

	DAY 8	DAY 9	DAY 10
WEIGHT TRAINING	20 minutes of Compound Exercise; Overload on Target Exercise	25 minutes of Compound Exercise; Overload on Target Exercise	30 minutes of Compound Exercise; Overload on Target Exercise
CARDIO TRAINING	No Cardio	No Cardio	No Cardio
NUTRITION	Moderate Fat, High Carb, High Protein	Moderate Fat, High Carb, High Protein	Moderate Fat, High Carb, High Protein

	DAY 11	DAY 12	DAY 13 AND 14
WEIGHT TRAINING	35 minutes of Compound Exercise;	40 minutes of Compound Exercise; Overload on Target Exercise	No Weights
CARDIO TRAINING	No Cardio	No Cardio	No Cardio
NUTRITION	Moderate Fat, High Carb, High Protein	Moderate Fat, High Carb, High Protein	Moderate Fat, High Carb, High Protein

See the Appendix or visit www.sportsworkout. com/muscleexplosioncharts for daily training & nutrition charts.

Week 3: Stretch-Pause Training

	DAY 15	DAY 16	DAY 17
WEIGHT TRAINING	Chest (3) Back (3) Biceps (2) Calves (2) Traps (1)	Shoulders (2) Triceps (2) Thighs/Quads (3) Hamstrings (2) Traps (1)	No Weights
CARDIO TRAINING	No Cardio	No Cardio	No Cardio
NUTRITION	Moderate Fat, High Carb, High Protein	Moderate Fat, High Carb, High Protein	Moderate Fat, High Carb, High Protein

	DAY 18	DAY 19	DAY 20 AND 21
WEIGHT TRAINING	Chest (3) Back (3) Biceps (2) Calves (2) Traps (1)	Shoulders (2) Triceps (2) Thighs/Quads (3) Hamstrings (2) Traps (1)	No Weights
CARDIO TRAINING	No Cardio	No Cardio	No Cardio
NUTRITION	Moderate Fat, High Carb, High Protein	Moderate Fat, High Carb, High Protein	Low Fat, Moderate Carb, High Protein

See the Appendix or visit www.sportsworkout. com/muscleexplosioncharts for daily training & nutrition charts.

Week 4: Stretch-Pause Training

	DAY 22	DAY 23	DAY 24
WEIGHT TRAINING	Chest (3) Back (3) Biceps (2) Calves (2) Traps (1)	Shoulders (2) Triceps (2) Thighs/Quads (3) Hamstrings (2) Traps (1)	No Weights
CARDIO TRAINING	No Cardio	No Cardio	No Cardio
NUTRITION	Moderate Fat, High Carb, High Protein	Moderate Fat, High Carb, High Protein	Moderate Fat, High Carb, High Protein

	DAY 25	DAY 26	DAY 27 AND 28
WEIGHT TRAINING	Chest (3) Back (3) Biceps (2) Calves (2) Traps (1)	Shoulders (2) Triceps (2) Thighs/Quads (3) Hamstrings (2) Traps (1)	No Weights
CARDIO TRAINING	No Cardio	No Cardio	No Cardio
NUTRITION	Moderate Fat, High Carb, High Protein	Moderate Fat, High Carb, High Protein	Low Fat, Moderate Carb, High Protein

See the Appendix or visit www.sportsworkout. com/muscleexplosioncharts for daily training & nutrition charts.

If you have completed the program once, you may start on Day 1 again without a break.

If this is your second round through the program without a break, take a FULL week off training before starting again. This is CRITICAL for recovery purposes.

How and Why the Program Works

Now that you've seen the "big picture," this section presents a more in-depth look at how the pieces fit together. This is an optional section but a good read if you want to really understand why it all works when combined and timed the way it is.

Also, understanding how each aspect of the program fits with the others to get the best results will allow you to make changes as you get more experienced with it.

The Nuts and Bolts of Week 1: Metabolic Acceleration and Tissue Remodeling Training

Week 1 is where we start pulling back the slingshot on your muscle growth. We use specific dietary and exercise techniques to basically deplete your body and set up the massive rebound in the next phase.

This week is based on low-carb eating to deplete the carbs in your body and lower your calorie intake. Your body will switch to fat-burning mode for one-and-a-half to two days. Throughout the week, you'll follow a very basic supplementation program of multivitamins and protein powder. You can also include glutamine after workouts (highly recommended). DO NOT take any creatine during this phase! We want to save it for the transition to the NEXT week, where you'll get the most bang for your buck with it.

Training on these first two days is "Metabolic Acceleration," using Fat Loss Circuit Training. This burns lots of calories, hastens the departure of carbs and water, and helps your body switch into fat-burning mode more quickly. You'll do total-body workouts on both days, increasing the number of sets on Day 2 while also decreasing "rest" time. All of this helps ramp up your metabolism.

Day 3 is a complete rest day to help you recover. Because this is a muscle-building program, we don't want to go TOO deeply into ketosis, a nutritional state in which your body burns ketones from fat metabolism for energy instead of glucose. Therefore, Day 3 is also a higher carb-eating day. This provides a nice anabolic burst. But here's the key: It's still a LOW CALORIE day (i.e., at least 500 calories below your personal maintenance calorie intake). This is the fat-loss phase after all!

On Day 4, go back to low-carb eating and perform Tissue Remodeling Training. I call this Lactic Acid Training, but with a very specific focus.

The training increases the body's lactic acid levels and keeps them elevated. This increases the level of growth hormone, a potent fat-burning, muscle-building hormone.

The exercises you'll use focus on the stretch and contracted positions of the target muscle group, using high reps and a partial range of motion. For example, for chest, you'll use dumbbell and keep the dumbbells in the stretched-wide position. Then you'll move to the top few inches of the bench press to hit the contracted position (with heavy weight and high reps). You'll finish with a single, full-range VERY HIGH rep set of an exercise for the target muscle group.

Two nutrient-isolation days follow. The first day focuses entirely on protein. You've been eating low carb and teaching your body to burn fat for energy. Suddenly depriving it of fat forces it to seek out the most convenient fat source: body fat.

The Interval Training, or alternating bouts of intense cardio training and rest periods, done on this day will encourage your body to use plenty of body fat for energy. The intervals are done completely on their own. They're not competing with the weight training days. The intervals done on this day should be challenging, but NOT full-on sprints. We want to get the cardio benefits of intervals but without hitting the body too hard. We don't want to compromise recovery for the training to come.

The second nutrient-isolation day is designed to create a desperate need for protein. This day, you eat only fruit.

Next week, when you eat plenty of protein, your body will aggressively store it in the form of muscle.

Because you will be staying away from protein, don't take glutamine on this day. Glutamine is an amino acid, a protein component. You will get plenty of it next week.

Don't train on this day either. You're depleting your body's free-circulating protein, but you don't want to excessively break down muscle tissue. Just that depletion will create a desperate need for protein.

An all-fruit day is very cleansing for the body, and a perfect switch from a high-protein, high-meat diet. Eat as much fruit as you want. Your body will stay busy absorbing the carbohydrates from the fruit. Be sure to drink plenty of water as well.

The Nuts and Bolts of Week 2: 5-Day Structural Attack

This week is pretty straightforward once you've gone through a couple of the workouts.

Basically, you're going to take one exercise and perform only that exercise the entire week, using a specialized training structure called Compound Exercise Overload. At its simplest, you take a weight with which you can perform six reps and perform three reps with it. Then rest 20 seconds, then go again. Rest 20 seconds. Go again. You repeat this until you can no longer perform three reps. When you get to this point, reduce the weight (by 10 or 20 pounds, depending on the exercise) and continue the three-rep sets. Continue this until your prescribed workout time is up.

The trick with this week is that every day you increase the time you use this technique. You also increase the starting weight for each workout (for at least the first three days). The first day, follow the technique for 20 minutes. The second day, make it 25 minutes. The third day, 30 minutes, etc. This forces an increase in workload and a SERIOUS body adaptation for the target exercise.

During this week it is CRITICAL to keep all demanding outside activities to a minimum. Do NO cardio this week, and work no other exercises or body parts. Period. We're looking for maximum adaptation to one single exercise.

As you start this week, you're coming off a week of low-calorie eating coupled with higher-rep training. You're also coming off an all-fruit day that has your body set up to store protein FAST. Put this all together and you're nutritionally PRIMED for maximum muscle growth.

In terms of nutrition, you want to be eating PLENTY of food this week, at least 1,500 to 2,000 calories more than maintenance levels. We're not looking for low-fat eating here. I still recommend that you do your best to eat healthy, minimally-processed foods that are as close to their natural state as possible. But DO NOT be afraid to eat some fat. It will give you calories and help raise your hormone production.

The Nuts and Bolts of Weeks 3 and 4: Stretch-Pause Training.

"During these two weeks, you'll continue with higher-calorie eating, or at least 1,000 calories more than maintenance levels. We're not following a strict diet here, but do eat reasonably. Keep junk foods to a minimum to keep fat gain under control. We're looking for relatively high-protein intake, along with plenty of carbs and moderate amounts of fat. (I'll spell out details in the Nutrition section.)

These two weeks, you'll also follow a specialized type of training I call Stretch-Pause Training. It's similar to Rest-Pause Training.

Stretch-Pause Training is a three-part set. The first part involves a full-range movement, for example, a barbell bench press.

The second part is a stretch-accentuated movement such as dumbbell flyes. Hold the stretch for a count of five to stretch out the muscle tissue and the fascia.

The third part is Partial-Range Training using the same exercise and weight you started the set with. This time, however, do only the top one-quarter of the range of motion while using a very concentrated and deliberate movement to really focus the contraction on the target muscles.

During the first week of this training, DO NOT use the specific exercise you used during the 5-Day Structural Attack. You'll do that exercise again during the SECOND week of this training, when you'll notice a BIG jump in strength.

During Weeks 2, 3, and 4, I don't list any specific cardio training. The reason is that I've packed it into Week 1, where it'll do you the most good and have the least detrimental effect on muscle growth. Cardio training takes energy, and we want your body's energy going into building new muscle tissue and recovery. But we don't neglect it at all, believe me. When you do squats and deadlifts in Week 2, you'll be getting a hard cardio workout. Don't think for a second that you're getting off easy.

The Sum of All Parts

As you can see, the training and nutrition of each week builds upon the last, making the whole greater than the sum of all parts. The synergistic effect of the various nutrient and training regimes allows you to effectively build muscle and strength by taking advantage of a very strict fat-loss phase.

You're basically slingshotting yourself forward in terms of muscle and strength. You pull yourself down with the fat-loss week, then rebound back up in subsequent weeks. This technique VERY effectively forces the body to build muscle and keeps body fat levels down at the same time!

Muscle Explosion Training Techniques

In this section, you'll learn in greater detail about each of the following specific training techniques. To get the most out of the program, read through each section so you understand how it all works.

Metabolic Acceleration

Tissue Remodeling

Interval Training

5-Day Structural Attack

Stretch-Pause Training

The Core Combo

These methods are incorporated into the program at very specific times, depending on the nutrients you are eating and the type of training that came before and will come after.

By using specific training methods at specific times, you greatly improve the results you can get. One thing sets up the next thing, which sets up the next thing, etc., to work with and maximize your body's metabolic capabilities.

Read through each section to be sure you understand what to do and why. The more you know and understand, the better you'll be able to adjust the training for your own body, and the more effective the Muscle Explosion Program will be.

A Note About WHEN to Train

Honestly, the best time to train for muscle mass and strength is whenever you are able to put the most effort into it AND can eat a very big meal soon afterward. It's no good training hard, then not being able to feed yourself after. You won't get the best result. That post-workout meal is absolutely CRITICAL to success.

Personally, I like to train in the late afternoon/early evening. This way, I'm able to eat a bit before training and still have time to finish with a big meal in the evening. When YOU feel best to train is totally up to you and your schedule.

Metabolic Acceleration

The first two training days of the Muscle Explosion Program involve what I call "Metabolic Acceleration." The goal here is twofold. First and most, we're looking to quickly ramp up the metabolism. Second, because we're doing low-carb eating, we want to use training that gets rid of the carbs in your body as quickly as possible.

To accomplish these goals, we use "Fat Loss Circuit Training."

Fat Loss Circuit Training is a technique I've developed primarily for losing fat quickly. Think of it as the first step toward pulling back on that metabolic slingshot as you aim for a massive muscle growth response. It ramps up the metabolism like crazy! It's simple once you get the hang of it, but it's one of the most demanding styles of fat-loss training you can do. The cardio component also helps you build up your cardiovascular system, which is important even when training for muscle mass.

To perform Fat Loss Circuit Training, you'll need access to weight training equipment, cardio equipment, and/or benches or stairs, preferably located in fairly close proximity to each other.

This is harder to do in a crowded gym, as you'll be moving quickly back and forth between different pieces of equipment. If someone hops on your cardio machine the moment you step off and you have to wait to get back on, you'll defeat the purpose of the workout. It's better to do this training in an uncrowded gym where you have more freedom to use equipment or, better yet, in a home gym with weights and cardio equipment and no one waiting for anything.

If you DO have to work out in a crowded gym, follow the alternate instructions described in the last two paragraphs of the Setup section. Do the training as weights first, then separate cardio immediately after.

How It Works

Essentially, this is combined circuit/interval training. You will be going back and forth between your weight training exercises and one cardio exercise for the duration of the workout. Your rest period for weights will be your cardio, and your rest period for cardio will be your weights. You will do your entire workout without any break.

This combination is very effective for a number of reasons:

- It forces your body to burn calories at a high level during the workout itself while greatly boosting your metabolism for a long time after.

- It strongly activates ALL the major energy systems in the body. The weights hit the Phosphocreatine system (for immediate bursts of energy), the Glycolytic system (for high-power but still immediate energy), and the Oxidative system (for longer-duration energy production). Typical training focuses on just one or two of these systems.

- It uses resistance and cardio training so you get all the benefits of both in one workout. The goal is maximum metabolic stimulation.

- It dramatically increases your metabolism, leading to increased fat burning long after the workout (more so than either weights or cardio alone).

- It saves time. You get both weights and cardio in the same amount of time as your regular workout.

- You're still able to use heavy weights in your weight training, helping to preserve muscle mass.

How to Do It

Step 1: Setup

For the most efficient workout possible, have most or all of your exercises pre-set and ready to go. The less time you spend on this during the workout itself, the more effective the workout will be, especially since you want to be continually active throughout the entire workout.

If you can't pre-set everything, choose exercises that have very little setup time—for example, dumbbell or cable exercises. You can use any type of cardio that is convenient and enjoyable to you, be it a machine, stair-stepping, or even skipping rope.

If you are working out in a crowded gym, try to claim an area for yourself and focus on dumbbell exercises. You won't have to wait in line for weight machines that way.

If you don't have access to convenient cardio machines, you're going to have go low-tech. You'll need to do stair-stepping (stepping up two stairs then back down works well), bench-stepping (step onto a flat bench or step platform, then back down), or rope-jumping (be sure you're not close to anyone if you choose this). These approaches work just as well as cardio machines and allow you to perform this training style in a busier setting.

Step 2: Warm-Up

Do a few minutes of low-intensity cardio as a warm-up. You may wish to do a few light sets of a few of the exercises you'll be working with. Don't tire yourself out; just get a light sweat going.

Step 3: Start with 40 seconds of moderate intensity cardio (on Day 2 of the program, it's 20 seconds)

This could mean setting the stair machine to a level that isn't easy but isn't so challenging that you exhaust yourself right away. Watch the timer on your machine and go for approximately 40 seconds. (I say approximately because there will generally be a slight lag time when you step on and off.) On Day 1, you'll be doing 40 seconds between weight sets. On Day 2, you'll be doing 20 seconds.

Many cardio machines have a "rest period" feature that lets you leave the machine on without erasing your program while you've stepped off. Normally, it's about two minutes. That should be enough time to complete your weight set. Treadmills will keep on moving when you step off. I recommend draping a towel over the console to let people know the machine is occupied so they don't jump on it without realizing it's moving.

Many machines also have a feature that runs you through a series of time periods. On the stair machine, I've found that if you set the session length for 20 minutes, you get a 40-second time period that's perfect for judging your cardio periods.

Step 4: Do a set of weights

Go as quickly as you can to your first exercise. Do a set of the first exercise on your program for the day. Do this with no rest, going immediately from the cardio to the weights. Do all your reps until you approach muscular failure–but don't meet or surpass that. Due to the high training volume we'll be doing, pushing to failure on every set will compromise muscle recovery.

So, maintain a do-or-die rep for every weight set, but stop one rep before it. You'll learn to know when it's coming.

Step 5: Go right back to the cardio

Get back on the treadmill and do another 40 seconds (or 20 seconds, if that's what you're on) of moderate-intensity cardio.

Step 6: Repeat the cycle for the duration of the workout

You will be going back and forth continuously between cardio and your weight training exercises, using the cardio as the rest period between your weight sets. Over the course of your workout, you'll be burning calories via cardio and weights AND working your muscles with intense, heavy weight training. It's tough training, but very effective!

When performing this training, you'll do ALL YOUR SETS FOR ONE BODY PART before moving on to the next. It will look like this:

40 seconds cardio

1 set of chest

40 seconds cardio

1 set of chest

40 seconds cardio

1 set of chest

40 seconds cardio

1 set of back

40 seconds cardio

1 set of back

40 seconds cardio

1 set of back

Repeat until all sets are done!

Notes:

1. Fat Loss Circuit Training can be used with nearly any form of cardio exercise as long as it is convenient to go back and forth to the weight regimen. The real key here is to maintain activity for the entire workout.

2. Work out for no more than 45 minutes when doing the Muscle Explosion Program. (The programs in this book are designed to stay below that time range.) Do any more than that and you will be breaking yourself down too much.

3. When you're working thighs during Fat Loss Circuit Training, be extra careful. Because most cardio activities work the legs, they aren't getting much recovery time between sets. There is no shame in holding on to solid objects for balance when you need to!

Doing Your Cardio Without Any Equipment: Stair/Bench-Stepping

If you aren't able to get on a cardio machine to do your 40 seconds (or 20 seconds) of training, try this instead: It's basic stair-stepping, and it works like a charm as a low-tech cardio exercise. Stand in front of some stairs. There should be at least two stairs that you can step up and down. A railing for balance is helpful for when you get fatigued. Be sure you have a clock or watch to keep track of your time. (You may need a partner to shout out times to you if your watch doesn't have a timer alarm.)

Step up and down the first two stairs for one or two minutes as a brief warm-up and to practice the pattern. The stepping pattern is as follows:

Right foot up on Step 1

Left foot up on Step 2

Right foot up on Step 2

Left foot down on Step 1

Right foot down on floor

Left foot down on floor

Repeat

Go through this pattern until you feel comfortable with it. It can be reversed by starting with the left foot on Step 1. Try both ways and do whichever is most comfortable to you. That's pretty much it. You can adjust your pace, going faster or slower in your stepping to adjust how difficult you want to make the cardio training. As you get in better shape, the stepping movement can turn into a hopping movement.

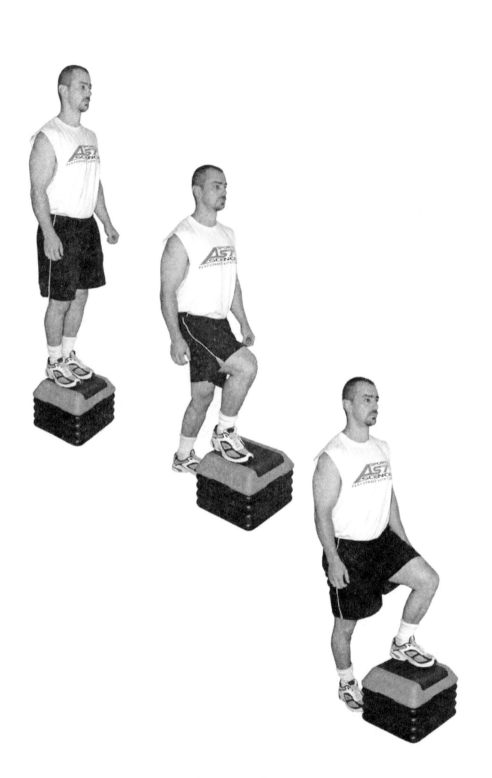

Stair/Bench-Stepping

TISSUE REMODELING TRAINING

Sure, the name "Tissue Remodeling" sounds painful. And to be honest, it's NOT going to be a comfortable experience. But it's THE most effective method I've found to literally pave the way for muscle growth. It's also an almost COMPLETELY NEGLECTED aspect of the muscle- and strength-building process. With it, you can UNLOCK your TRUE muscle-growth potential. Because you know what? Muscle development is NOT all genetics. A lot of it comes down to your basic physiology, much of which can be QUICKLY IMPROVED through proper training.

It involves specialized training techniques that prepare your physiology for future muscle growth.

After all, you would never build a house without first pouring a foundation and framing it out with two-by-fours to create a solid structure. And you wouldn't put up the drywall for the rooms without first installing the ventilation, electrical, and plumbing, would you?

But that's what many people do when using "standard" muscle-building training. They start putting up the drywall (muscle tissue) without making sure they have enough ventilation, electrical, and plumbing to fully support it.

You don't see many people reinforcing the deep structures of the body (the connective tissue) to REALLY maximize growth and strength. THIS is where "Tissue Remodeling Training" comes in.

Part 1: Foundation and Frame

The first step to prepare your body for future muscle and strength improvements is to work on your foundation and frame, which is your connective tissue. Connective tissue consists of tendons (which connect muscles to bones), ligaments (which connect bones to bones), and fascia (a "pillowcase" of tough tissue that keeps the muscles in place).

Connective tissue is what holds your body together and gives it structure and support. Without it, you couldn't move, and you certainly couldn't move any sort of weight at all!

But the VAST majority of training programs don't address connective tissue. That is a HUGE mistake because connective tissue is where the REAL strength in your body originates. Muscles can actually gain strength and size quite quickly but are often limited by connective tissue strength, which develops more slowly.

Take the steroid user, for example. What happens when a steroid user gets bigger muscles really fast? The muscles can bench press 500 pounds, but the tendons can only handle 400 pounds. SNAP. Not a good thing!

If we focus on preparing the connective tissue for heavier workloads, we will give the muscles a much greater base upon which to build strength. You'll be building a strong "foundation and frame" of tendons and ligaments. (I'll talk more on fascia below.)

This "foundation and frame" training requires what I call Partial Training. Partial Training is simple. You take your normal, everyday exercises and do them only in a very short, very specific range of motion.

1. It allows you to use much heavier loads than you normally could over a full range of motion. For example, you can bench press a LOT more in the top two inches of the exercise than you can over the whole range of motion.

2. It focuses more work on a specific point in the range of motion. A good example is the stretch position of the dumbbell flye. The most effective part of the exercise is the bottom stretch position. You can't use as much weight when you do partials at the bottom, but you are focusing on a very powerful point in the range of motion.

In Tissue Remodeling, we're going to work on BOTH of these advantages while also eliminating two of the biggest DISADVANTAGES of heavy Partial Training.

What are those disadvantages?

When you do heavy Partial Training, as great as it is for developing connective tissue, your sets last only a VERY short time. It doesn't take long to press a bar two inches, then lower it back down. You can do a set of five or six reps in about 15 seconds.

This puts a great strength-building load on the connective tissue but doesn't draw much blood flow into the area. And blood flow is CRITICAL for developing your connective tissue quickly.

Connective tissue has a notoriously poor blood supply. Ask anyone who's had a tendon or ligament injury. He or she will tell you it took a long time to fully heal! Normal low-rep Partial Training doesn't force much blood into the connective tissue. But HIGH-REP Partial Training DOES.

So instead of doing five or six reps for our Partials, we're going to do 30+ rep sets (at least on the first sets—more on that in a minute). This solves the problem of blood supply. It also solves the second big disadvantage: "time under tension" for the muscles.

Time under tension is basically a measure of how long a muscle has resistance placed on it, or how long it has to contract. So if a set lasts 60 seconds and the muscle is under tension the entire time, that's 60 seconds of time under tension. It's a useful measure for determining how effective a training technique or exercise is at promoting muscle growth. Ideally, for muscle growth, you want to achieve 30 to 60 seconds of time under tension.

As I mentioned above, normal Partial Training takes just 15 seconds to do five or six reps. Not much time under tension there. By doing high rep Partial Training, you achieve time under tension upwards of 30 seconds to a minute—which is ideal for producing muscle growth. So, you get connective tissue training AND stimulate muscle growth while using heavier-than-normal weights.

Now we come to fascia, the fibrous pillowcases around your muscles that keep them in place in your body.

Fascia has both positives and negatives when it comes to muscle and strength. Without fascia, your muscles would flop around all over, and your contractions would be ineffective. In fact, when fascia is injured, muscle contraction and movement are impaired. Fascia is a critical facet of your body's connective tissue makeup.

But there's the major negative. Tight fascia can restrict muscle growth. Tight fascia can be a significant reason people don't see muscle growth when they're doing just about everything else right. When the muscle has no room to grow, it just can't grow.

What can do we do about that?

We're going to use high-rep Partials to "wiggle" the fascia and force it to expand. We're going to alternate Partials in the CONTRACTED position of a body part (this helps fill the muscles with blood) with partials in the maximum STRETCH position of a body part (this helps expand the fascia after the muscle is filled with blood).

Think of it this way: When your clothes come out of the dryer, they feel a bit smaller than when you last wore them, right? Think of that pair of tighter jeans as your fascia. What do you do to loosen up those jeans? You put them on, then squat up and down a few times to get them to stretch a bit and expand, giving you a little more room in them. Same thing with a tight shirt. You put it on and then pull on it here and there to stretch the material and make it a bit looser.

That is EXACTLY what we're going to do with your fascia. By alternating the partial movements in the two extreme positions of the muscle, we're going to give your muscles a little bit more room inside, and THAT means room to GROW.

One side note, and I'll get into this in the Supplementation section: I HIGHLY recommend taking a joint support supplement while doing the entire Muscle Explosion Program. Your body needs the raw materials to help support and rebuild from the connective tissue-targeted training we're doing. To keep your joints in good shape and well lubricated, joint supplements are critical.

Part 2: Ventilation, Electrical, and Plumbing

Now that we've addressed the foundation and frame, it's time to focus on the guts of our house/body: ventilation, electrical, and plumbing. Let's look at ventilation and plumbing first.

For our purposes, ventilation and plumbing can be compared to blood vessels (which are definitely plumbing) and the nutrients and oxygen carried in the blood (which we'll call ventilation). They're very much related, so I'll talk about them together.

If you've been training awhile, you know you have certain muscle groups that don't pump up easily and some that pump up like crazy—even if you're just carrying groceries to the car. The parts that pump up easily, I can almost guarantee you, are the body parts that GROW easily, too.

So what's the connection? Blood circulation.

The blood supply to a muscle has a direct connection to how easily that muscle grows AND how quickly it recovers from training. Nutrients and oxygen are supplied by the blood, and nutrients and oxygen are necessary to rebuild and repair muscle cells. Without a steady stream of both, growth and recovery are blunted. They'll still happen, just not as quickly or efficiently.

Also of critical importance is the removal of waste products. Before recovery can take place, you have to get rid of the junk (specifically the metabolic junk left over from muscle damage as a result of training).

When you look through the program in the Appendix, you may notice, a "+2" in the sets listed on Tissue Remodeling Training. Those are two very high rep sets done at the tail end of each body part, AFTER the back and forth Partial Training. The primary purpose of these high-rep sets is to improve your plumbing and ventilation.

Very high rep training increases what is called "capillarization" of the muscle tissue. To explain it, I'll go back to a little basic physiology. I'll keep things simple.

In your body, veins and arteries make up your circulatory system. Blood gets pumped through your circulatory system by the heart, stopping by the lungs to pick up oxygen and expel carbon dioxide, and stopping by the digestive system to pick up nutrients and get rid of waste.

The good stuff has to get transferred to the body's cells, but the bigger blood vessels are too big to do it effectively. So the circulatory system gets smaller. The arteries (that carry the blood when it's full of nutrients and oxygen) scale down and down until they're just big enough for one or two red blood cells to get through. It's in these little blood vessels that all the "action" happens. These little blood vessels are called "capillaries."

In the capillaries, oxygen gets into the cells and carbon dioxide gets picked up to be transported away. Nutrients also get transferred to the cells, and waste products get picked up to be transported out. Back to our house analogy, it's like the door through which you bring in the groceries and take out the trash, only a whole lot smaller.

What's the point of all this?

The more capillaries you have, the MORE nutrients and oxygen you can get into your muscle cells. When your muscles get more food and oxygen, they recover faster [Reference 19] and have the potential to grow larger FASTER.

With very high rep training, you're giving yourself better plumbing and ventilation by increasing the number and

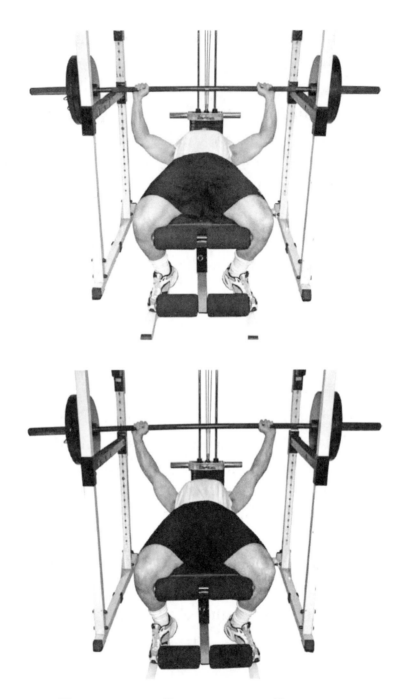

EXAMPLE OF CONTRACTED-POSITION
PARTIAL BENCH PRESS

density of the capillaries in your muscles. [Reference 18] You're basically setting the stage for future muscle growth by improving the blood supply to the muscles. That's the point of doing very high rep training.

Think about what I said at the start of this section. The muscles that pump up easily are the muscles that have a good blood supply and generally grow more easily. This training is targeted to improve the blood supply to ALL muscles.

The only hitch with training to increase capillary density is that you're using light weights for high reps which, on its own, doesn't build muscle. It primarily works Type 1 muscle fibers, which are targeted for endurance. Therefore, the brief duration of this training (two days) is a compromise between increasing capillary density and working against ourselves in terms of muscle building. If you REALLY wanted to focus on increasing capillary density, a training program of three to four weeks of very high rep training would improve the effect (but at the cost of backing way off on the higher-tension, lower rep training that's most effective for building muscle.).

Each time you go through this program and do the very high rep training, you're going to improve your capillary density a little bit more—without taking a big hit on your overall muscle-building.

So what about your electrical system?

Well, that's an added bonus of this very high rep training. Your nervous system (a.k.a. your electrical system) can be trained to produce faster impulses to get faster contraction out of the muscles, thus improving power. Power is a mix of strength AND speed; you need BOTH to produce maximum power.

Speed training with lighter weights is a KEY component of the programs of top powerlifters. They train VERY heavy to develop the muscles and connective tissue, and they train LIGHT and with maximum speed to train the nervous system to fire more efficiently. If you're using only heavy weights, the nervous system simply doesn't get the same degree of speed training.

That's where the very high rep sets also serve a dual purpose. Not only are we doing high reps, we're doing them VERY FAST! This is speed training, and it can help train your nerves to fire more explosively. You're using light weight and cranking out the reps pretty much as fast as you can. This pumps a lot of blood into the muscles, which forces the increase in capillarization AND tunes the nervous system to fire explosively.

How to Do Tissue Remodeling Training

The first part of Tissue Remodeling Training (the back and forth between contracted-position Partials and stretch-position Partials that I described above) is done using a technique I call Lactic Acid Training. In a nutshell, this style of training is designed to force your body to produce a lot of lactic acid in the target muscles and keep it there by utilizing high reps and very short rest periods.

Research has shown that the presence of lactic acid, a metabolic byproduct of energy production in the muscles, which lowers the acidity of the bloodstream when it accumulates, can cause an increase in both growth hormone and testosterone secretion [Reference 1, 2, 7, 9]. These are two of the most anabolic (muscle building) and lipolytic (fat burning) hormones in the human body!

The result? Your body is forced to build muscle while burning tremendous amounts of fat. Here are some additional benefits of Lactic Acid Training as done with this program (you're going to LOVE these!):

The release of growth hormone is facilitated and enhanced by low/stable insulin levels. The two hormones simply don't function well together. By performing Lactic Acid Training on the days when your insulin levels are low—two days of the low-carb diet phase, for example—you will maximize the effect of this training style on your growth hormone levels. You'll basically get the most bang for your Lactic Acid Training buck.

Lactic Acid Training causes your muscles to fail not due to contractile failure (the point at which your muscle fibers are too fatigued to continue) but because of lower cellular pH. The acid lowers pH, which is the acid-base balance in the blood. When it gets too low, your muscles are unable to contract effectively. Not being able to push to contractile failure protects the muscles from excessive breakdown, which is critical to preserving muscle mass under the reduced-calorie conditions of this specific week.

Lactic Acid Training also burns quite a lot of calories during the session itself. This is because of the very short rest periods and high volume of work. This, in turn, keeps your heart rate in an aerobic conditioning zone even during rest, further increasing the benefits of the training.

The short rest periods and focused volume deliver a huge pump, even under the low-calorie, low-hydration, and low-glycogen conditions you're operating under in this week of the program.

Increased growth hormone levels also increase the use of fat for energy during recovery after intense exercise. This means your body will be burning fat to help you recover from your training [Reference 2].

High-rep Lactic Acid Training also trains the Type 1 muscle fibers (endurance-oriented), developing and multiplying the cellular energy furnaces known as mitochondria that rely on fats to supply energy to your cells. This means your body will become more productive at burning fat, even while at rest.

The high volume of training you will be doing will also help stimulate growth hormone production [References 6, 8]. Higher training volume has been shown to produce a better growth hormone response than lower volume training.

Put all of these amazing benefits together and you've got one incredibly powerful training technique by itself. Now put EVERYTHING I've talked about together and you're going to experience the power of Tissue Remodeling Training.

How to Perform Lactic Acid Training

The basic execution of Lactic Acid Training for this program is very simple.

1. Pick one single exercise, using a weight you can handle for 20 to 50 reps—remember, in our case we'll be working only the TOP few inches of the CONTRACTED-position range of motion of an exercise, the top few inches of the bench press, for example. You may have to experiment with weights to determine the proper load. Generally speaking, you can probably work with a weight that is 80

percent to 100 percent of your one rep max, depending on the exercise. With partial squats and bench presses, you can most likely manage even more than that for high reps.

2. Do as many reps as you can until your muscles are burning so strongly and are so flooded with lactic acid that you can't move the weight. You will probably have to drop the weight pretty quickly by this point!

3. Rest 20 seconds.

4. Now go immediately into the STRETCH-position partial exercise. Examples of stretch-position exercises for each muscle group are listed below. Do 20 to 30 or more reps in ONLY the stretch position of the exercise.

Stretch-Position Exercises

Chest - dumbbell flyes

Back - stiff-arm pushdowns or dumbbell pullovers

Quads - sissy squats

Hamstrings - stiff-legged deadlifts

Biceps - incline dumbbell curls

Triceps - overhead dumbbell tricep extensions

Calves - donkey calf raises (or any calf raise with a focus on the stretch portion)

Shoulders - cable laterals

5. Rest 20 seconds.

6. Now do another set with the same weight of the contracted-position exercise. Examples of contraction-position exercises for each muscle group are listed below. You will probably be able to do only eight to 10 reps with that weight, even if you just did 50 reps a minute ago. The short rest period means the lactic acid hasn't had time to fully clear, so you will fail due to lactic acid build-up in the muscles rather than true muscular failure (which is what we want here).

    Contraction-Position Exercises

    Chest - barbell bench press

    Back - deadlifts, chin-ups, or any rowing variation

    Quads - squats

    Hamstrings - leg curls

    Biceps - barbell curls

    Triceps - weighted dips or close grip bench press

    Calves - standing or seated calf raises

    Shoulders - barbell shoulder press

7. Rest 20 seconds, then do another set of the stretch-position exercise.

8. Repeat this for a total of six to eight sets per body part, depending on the program requirements and which

body part you're working. If the program calls for eight sets, that means you'll do four sets of each exercise, alternated with each other.

The number of reps you can do may drop to five or less, but don't worry. Rep numbers are not particularly important here. You are trying to churn out as much lactic acid as possible, and the 20-second rest is not enough time for the body to clear it away. But it is enough time to allow you to go again soon. You are likely to find, after a few sets, that you hit a steady state where you get about the same number of reps on each set.

One thing to note: The negative, or eccentric, aspect of the rep (generally the lowering of the weight) need not be emphasized when doing Lactic Acid Training. Research has shown that the positive or concentric phase of the rep (when the muscle is contracting) is more productive in terms of growth hormone release [Reference 4] than the negative phase.

This doesn't mean you should ignore the negative—just don't focus on it to the detriment of the positive aspect, especially when doing these high-rep, partial sets. In plain English, it is better to focus on getting more reps than on doing slow negatives.

Notes:

1. Have your two exercises set up and ready to go before you launch into the repetitions for that body part.

2. Lactic Acid Training is hard to do with a partner because you may rest too long between sets. Twenty seconds usually isn't enough time to switch places, do a set and switch places again, especially if you have to change weights between sets.

3. If you work with a partner with similar strength levels, try it this way: You start with your set of the contracted-position partial exercise. Rest your 20 seconds, then do your stretch exercise. When you start your stretch exercise, your partner starts his/her contracted position exercise. When you're done, your partner is done and you switch. Then you go back and forth between the two exercises for the designated number of sets.

4. Have a water bottle handly when doing Lactic Acid Training. The rest periods are not long enough to go to a water fountain. The effectiveness of the training will be diminished considerably if you take too long getting a drink.

How to Perform Very High Rep Training

Once you've finished the Lactic Acid Training for your target body part, take a one minute rest to get set up for VERY High Rep Training. I recommend using the same exercise you used for the contract-position partials, but with a MUCH lighter weight. You can certainly use a different exercise, or you can use a variation of the previous exercise if it's easier to set up.

You want to select a weight that is VERY light. Something you normally wouldn't be caught dead training with is a good place to start.

To give you a frame of reference, I use 315 pounds on the contracted-position partials for bench press, then I drop the weight and use 95 pounds for the full-range, very-high-rep sets that follow. When doing barbell shoulder press, I use just the empty bar (same for barbell curls).

Check your ego at the door. That's not what we're working on now. You MUST use a weight that will allow you to get 30 (preferably more) reps on these sets for them to be really effective in improving the capillarization of the muscles.

Use a FAST movement for these reps. You want to focus on speed at the beginning of the sets. As you keep going, you'll start to get lactic acid build-up and your reps will slow down. Keep forcing out as many more reps as you can!

Close your eyes and really dig into the target muscles to squeeze every last ounce of movement out of them. By the time you hit the last reps, you should be struggling like the weight is your maximum lift, even if you've just finished your 58th rep!

This forcing of reps will help produce that capillarization of the muscles that gives you that base to build fresh, new muscle in the coming weeks. Now set the weight down, rest one minute, and do it again!

Interval Training

I'll lay it out for you: Interval Training is simply THE most efficient type of cardio you can perform. You can get pretty much ALL the benefits of longer-duration cardio but without the long duration. You don't get the boredom, you don't spend all your time doing it, and you don't have nearly the risk of overuse injuries.

I'm not going to get into too much detail about why Interval Training is superior, not only timewise but in terms of fat burning as well. Here it is in a nutshell:

Low-intensity exercise is defined as working at a heart rate of about 60 percent to 65 percent of your maximum heart rate (equal to 220 minus your age; thus, if you are 20 years old, 220 minus 20 is 200 maximum heart rate).

High-intensity exercise is defined as working at about 75 percent to 85 percent or more of your maximum heart rate. Using the example of 200 as your maximum heart rate, working at 60 percent of it would be 120 beats per minute. Eighty percent would be 160 beats per minute.

Let's crunch some numbers to show you exactly what I mean when I say high-intensity exercise burns more fat.

- Low-intensity training burns about 50 percent fat for energy while high-intensity training burns about 40 percent fat for energy. This is not a huge difference.

- Say, for example, that walking for 20 minutes burns 100 calories. Then 50 percent of 100 calories is 50 fat calories burned.

- Now say 10 minutes of Interval Training at a high intensity burns 160 calories. Forty percent of 160 calories is 64 fat calories burned.

- By doing the high-intensity work, you've just burned 14 more fat calories in half the time. Starting to sound good? There's more.

Low-intensity exercise only burns calories while you are actually exercising. That means the moment you stop exercising, your caloric expenditure falls to nearly baseline levels. Within minutes, you are not burning many more calories than if you hadn't done anything at all.

High-intensity exercise, on the other hand, continues to boost your metabolism long after you are done—often up to 24 hours after, depending on the length and intensity of the training session. This means you are continuing to burn many more calories all day long!

Low-intensity exercise does nothing to build or support muscle mass. Maintaining muscle mass is critical to an effective fat-loss strategy because muscle burns fat even at rest. Want to keep your metabolism working to burn fat? Do whatever you can to build or keep your muscle tissue. That's definitely the goal with this program!

High-intensity exercise has the potential to increase muscle mass. Compare the bodies of a top sprinter and a top marathon runner. The sprinter carries far more muscle mass. You won't get big muscles from high-intensity training on its own but, from a physiological standpoint, high-intensity training is fairly similar to weight training when it comes to body response.

How We're Going to Do Interval Training in this Program

Interval Training is based on a very simple concept: Go fast, then go slow. Repeat. It sounds easy, but within this simple formula are a tremendous number of possible variations and strategies you can employ to take full advantage of the power available to you.

Interval Training can be performed on almost any cardiovascular machine (treadmill, stair machine, stationary bike, elliptical trainer, etc.), as well as with almost any type of cardiovascular exercise (cycling, swimming, running, etc.).

Though the most convenient approach is to use time as a measure for intervals, you can also very easily use distance as your guide. For example, you can sprint between two telephone poles, then walk to the next one. You can sprint the length of a football field, then walk the width. You can even run up a flight of stairs then walk back down. The variations are truly endless!

Here's a quick rundown of different types of Interval Training, with the type YOU'LL be doing appearing LAST.

1. Aerobic Interval Training

This type involves relatively long work periods and shorter rest periods. Work periods are to be alternated with rest for the duration of the training. Work periods are generally two to five minutes long. The idea is to work at a speed that challenges you to make it to the end of that work interval. Your two-minute interval pace is, therefore, going to be significantly faster than your five-minute interval pace. The rest interval lasts 30 seconds to a minute. Naturally, the shorter the rest period, the tougher the training will be. Too much rest allows your body to recover too much, lessening the overall training effect of the exercise.

2. Maximal High-Intensity Intervals

This type of Interval Training is VERY high intensity and VERY effective for fat loss and cardio training. You essentially push yourself to the maximum on every single work interval you do!

It is extremely effective when training for sports that require all-out repeated efforts, such as football, soccer, hockey, etc.

If you want to get faster and recover faster, this is the training for you. Maximal Intervals are much shorter than Aerobic Intervals. Generally, the longest you'll be able to perform a maximal effort is about 30 seconds, so all the work intervals are 30 seconds or less.

Rest periods can be short or long, depending on what kind of shape a person is in and/or how much he or she wants to recover between intervals. Shorter rest periods make the work intervals more challenging, but the speed of the work will also drop quickly after a few intervals. Longer rest periods allow the body to recover a little more, allowing for faster speeds on more intervals. Rest periods should always be at least as long as the work periods to allow enough recovery to be able to perform well on the next work period.

3. Fartlek Training

Translated from Swedish, "fartlek" means "speed play." What is it? It's simple: fartlek Training is every type of interval rolled into one workout. You can start by jogging for five minutes, then walk for 30 seconds, then sprint for 30 seconds, then walk again, then run fast for two minutes and so on. The idea is to train at a wide variety of speeds, distances, and times to hit the widest variety of training parameters. This is an excellent way to keep your cardio interesting. You never have to do the same thing twice. This workout can last anywhere from 15 to 40 minutes, depending on the intensity at which you are working.

4. Sub-Maximal High-Intensity Intervals: This Is What You Will Be Doing on Day 6

Sub-Maximal Intervals are excellent for burning fat and building your cardiovascular conditioning, which is our goal on Day 6. We want to get in some good cardio training, but we're NOT trying to push so hard that we take a hit on recovery ability.

This type of Interval Training is very similar in concept and execution to Maximal Interval style. The difference: Instead of pushing yourself as hard as you can on each work interval, you work at a pace somewhat below your max. This allows you to do more total work intervals during the session while still keeping your intensity levels reasonably high.

Most interval programs on cardio machines follow this principle. The resistance/speed is increased to a higher level for a set time period, then reduced for a set time period. The level is not so high that you must put your maximum effort into each work interval, but it is at a level you could not keep up for long periods.

In this case, you're going to do 15 minutes of total cardio training time, alternating 30 seconds of work with 30 seconds at a very slow pace.

Your work level should be at about 80 percent to 90 percent of what you could do for a full-on maximum level for 30 seconds. Therefore, if your maximum is level 10 on the treadmill for 30 seconds, set your work interval to between eight and nine. You'll be doing 15 work intervals with 15 rest intervals.

Notice that on this training day, you're doing the Core Combo AFTER the cardio training. Because the cardio is only 15 minutes, I've taken the Core Combo out of the Tissue Remodeling Training days and added it here. Use the exercises listed in the Core Combo section, especially the abdominal exercises. They are designed to develop core strength and stability, which will come in handy as you start lifting heavier weights.

When you complete the Core Combo, feel free to perform some general stretching for your entire body. Everything is all warmed up, and the shorter overall workout time means you won't be too trashed to get in some good stretching.

5. Near-Maximal Aerobic Intervals: This Is What You MAY Be Doing Instead of Fat Loss Circuit Training

This form of Interval Training basically combines Aerobic Interval Training with Maximal Interval Training to allow you to work at near-peak levels for long periods. This has the benefit of burning a tremendous amount of calories for longer periods of work time than is possible with normal intervals.

You will use this cardio training style on the first two days of the program if you can't perform the regular Fat Loss Circuit Training in your gym due to crowded conditions or gym regulations. If so, you'll do all your weight sets first (with 30 seconds of rest between sets), then do a session of THIS style of cardio training. It's VERY effective for boosting the metabolism as well.

With this training, the work intervals themselves are short, but the rest periods are much shorter! Instead of pushing yourself to the max on every interval, you work at a pace somewhat short of your max. This allows you to perform near your max for longer periods of time. It is a very challenging form of Interval Training.

Here's how it works

Start with a work interval of 20 seconds and a rest interval of five seconds. Set a pace that you can keep up for only about one to two minutes before needing to stop.

Do that pace for 20 seconds, then go very slowly for five seconds. Then repeat this cycle for another 20 and five seconds. Keep repeating for a designated period of time, for example, five minutes, 10 minutes, or 15 minutes.

This type of training works well with cardio machines that allow you to switch resistance instantly or very quickly (stationary bikes, stair machines, or elliptical trainers often allow this). Machines that must cycle slowly through their speeds as they change do not work well. (Treadmills fall into this category.) You can also do this by running then walking, cycling then pedaling slowly, or even swimming hard then stroking lazily. You'll find it very challenging to constantly restart your momentum from scratch on every interval.

Please note: It's very important that you don't stop completely when you take your short rest period. Keep yourself moving, even if you're moving VERY slowly.

5-Day Structural Attack

What Is It?

It's an ominous sounding name. By the time you're finished, you're probably going to think it doesn't sound ominous enough.

But let me tell you, the results you're going to see in these five short days could very well surpass what you've seen in the last five MONTHS. It's that good. And it's that tough.

Basically, you're going to train using just ONE exercise for five workout days in a row. You're going to be training this single exercise with HEAVY weight and EXTREMELY high volume. Don't worry; I also include instructions on how to modify this five-day attack if you're not able to complete the five days in a row.

The reason we use only one exercise? More efficient and extremely rapid adaptation. To really maximize strength gains, the training is going to tell the body it needs to get good at ONE SINGLE MOVEMENT. Nothing else. When faced with this type of very specific stimulus, the body is capable of extraordinary adaptation. Your body will become its function, and that function will be coping with the single exercise you're doing for five days straight.

To give you an idea of how well this technique has worked for me, in testing the program with the deadlift I began deadlifting 365 pounds for three rep sets on Day 1. By the fourth day, I began the training session deadlifting 425 pounds for the same three rep sets. In only four days of constant, high-volume, very specific work, I ADDED 60 pounds to my deadlifting capability! I also went from weighing 202 pounds to weighing 209 pounds in just five days.

I believe the technical term for this is INSANE RESULTS.

Hyperplasia Anyone?

After using it on a number of muscle groups, I believe this technique has the potential to not only wake up dormant muscle fibers, but also to stimulate hyperplasia (muscle-fiber splitting to increase fiber number). These only happen with extreme tension and volume, which you will get here.

Actually confirming this would require muscle biopsies and counting muscle fibers (not really practical), but studies on cats and birds have shown hyperplasia when subjected to extreme stresses and tension. This five-day overload will take your muscle fibers right to the EDGE. When you combine this training with the TREMENDOUS flood of water and nutrients into the muscle cells that you're getting from the carb and creatine loading, you're looking at a training style that, in my opinion, has SERIOUS potential to achieve hyperplasia.

You are basically going to be stressing your fluid-saturated muscle cells to the point where, to keep up with the demands you're placing on them, they (in theory, of course) HAVE to split in order to cope.

What about training to failure?

When you're doing this training, you are going to AVOID MUSCULAR FAILURE. You will get close, but you will stay away from actually reaching it. This allows you to work with greater resistance for longer periods of time (greater volume). This also ensures that we avoid CHEMICAL MUSCLE FAILURE (failure due to lactic acid and other metabolic byproduct build-up and/or depleted cellular energy/ATP).

By staying away from chemical muscle failure, we allow for strong FIBER FATIGUE, which is a whole different ballgame. Your muscles won't fail because your body's pH is too low (from the acidity of lactic acid build-up), or because ATP (your basic energy molecule) stores are depleted. Your muscle fibers will be worked to their full capacity WITHOUT being stopped by that.

This training will take pretty much ALL the muscle fibers in the target muscle group to exhaustion and make sure they ALL get sufficiently damaged to stimulate growth. It's this extreme demand on your body that is going to give you extreme results.

The Plan of the Attack

The basis of the 5-Day Structural Attack phase is a technique I've developed and call Compound Exercise Overload. The first time you do this program, I HIGHLY recommend you do one of two exercises: squats or deadlifts.

Why just these two exercises? Why not bench press or barbell curls?

Because the squat and the deadlift are THE most effective overall mass- and strength-building exercises you can do. No question about it.

To maximize the overall effect of this technique in terms of body strength and muscle, YOU WILL GET THE BEST RESULTS using one of these two exercises. It's not going to be easy. In fact, I'm quite sure you'll be cursing me as you go through it. But you will LOVE the results you get. The squat or the deadlift attack your body's structure at its most basic level, building a foundation of strength that will make you downright UNSTOPPABLE when you get done.

The ONLY reason to use a different exercise the first time through is if you do not have much experience with either squats or deadlifts, or if you have an injury that prevents you from performing either exercise with good form.

The second time through, you can choose bench press or a different exercise. I WOULD recommend you choose an exercise that targets the upper body. It's a tough technique, and it's a good idea to alternate upper and lower body training to not completely overload either one.

Avoid doing this technique with any exercise that involves momentum or high skill, for example, exercises like power cleans or pulls. The force of momentum on the joints in these exercises doesn't lend itself to high-volume training. Also, as you get tired, your form will break down, especially on high-skill exercises like power cleans. That risks injury AND teaches and reinforces bad form, which is NOT what we want to do.

You CAN use this technique with isolation exercises, even though it's called Compound Exercise Overload. I've used the technique with dumbbell flyes on the Swiss Ball and with barbell curls with excellent results. But save those for the second (or later) round through the program. Like I said, choose squats or deadlifts the first time through.

When you do those squats and deadlifts, wear solid-soled shoes or boots. This will help minimize any loss of power into the squishiness of normal running shoes.

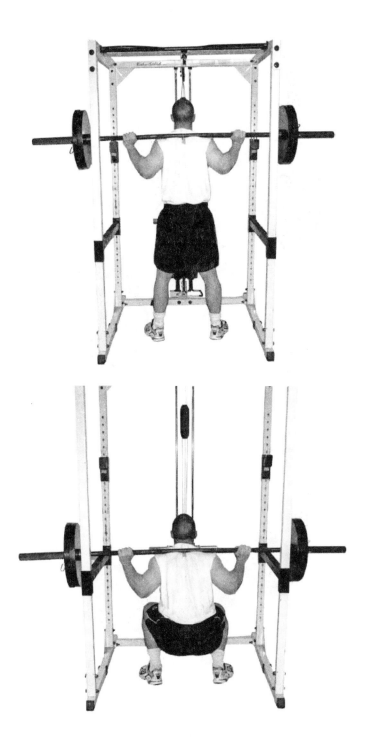

SQUATS

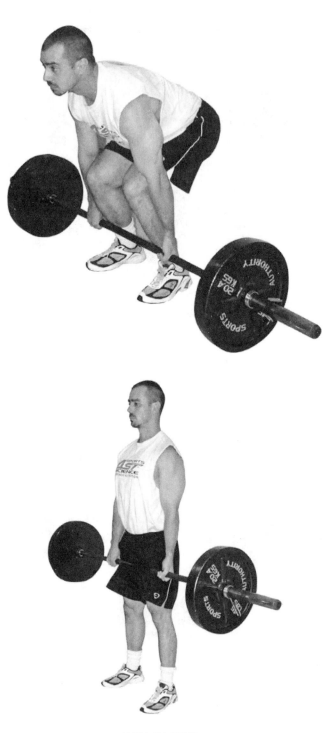

DEADLIFTS

Here's another helpful tip: Take 1,000 mg of Vitamin C about 45 minutes before the workout. This will minimize muscle soreness (and it WILL happen). Do this before EVERY training session this week!

The Compound Exercise Overload Technique

You're going to take a single compound exercise and do ONLY that exercise for the ENTIRE WORKOUT.

But that's not the brutal part.

The brutal part is that you are allowed only 30 seconds of rest between sets. (You'll get just 20 seconds when you use this technique with exercises other than the squat or deadlift.)

This is one of the toughest workouts you can do (when you do it right), but you WILL be rewarded with results. You're going to do it five days in a row, increasing the workout time EVERY SINGLE DAY.

This program really becomes about basic survival for your muscles.

Your body will use a tremendous emergency response to cope with this onslaught of steadily increasing training volume. We're going to go BEYOND typical soreness and muscular exhaustion. Your body will almost literally become a MACHINE at the specific exercise you're doing.

Here's a VERY IMPORTANT GUIDELINE: Do NOTHING else that is physically demanding this week, if you can help it at all. We don't want to confuse the body with ANY other stimulus. This means NO cardio, no abdominal training, no other body part worked in any way, shape, or form. I would even avoid heavy manual labor if you have the option. This will really help streamline the recovery process.

Compound Exercise Overload works to increase strength in several ways:

1. It focuses your nervous system on a single specific exercise, "greasing the groove" at a specific rep range. No competing training stimuli here, just very specific focus. This is one of the reasons Olympic lifters use only a few lifts in their training. It's also one of the reasons they can lift such extraordinary amounts of weight.

2. It allows you to have a LOT of practice lifting heavy weight. This helps you perfect your form and become more efficient with your lifting technique.

3. The high volume of training creates an emergency situation in your body that forces rapid adaptation by your body (both in muscle and connective tissue).

4. The high volume also forces a tremendous amount of blood into the target muscle group, which helps drive nutrients into those muscles, which helps them recover and grow!

Combine these four factors and you've got one POWERFUL workout.

How to Do It

First, select a compound exercise to work with, either the squat or the deadlift. The deadlift is a good choice because you won't have anybody bugging you because you're hogging a machine or power rack for the whole workout. If you do deadlifts, however, you MUST know what you're doing and have very good form when doing them. You're going to be doing a LOT of sets, and any form errors will be amplified over the course of the workouts.

If you're more comfortable with squats, do squats.

This training style is best done at a time when your gym is not crowded. You're going to be hogging a single exercise area for the entire workout. This isn't a big deal with deadlifts as you're using just a barbell. It might be trickier with the squat rack, but it will definitely be tougher on a bench press station (those always seem to have a line). If and when you DO use the bench press, I'd recommend doing them in the rack and using a moveable flat bench.

You won't be in the way as much, AND you'll be a lot safer when training.

Do a warm-up before getting started. Whatever you prefer for a warm-up is fine. I like to do some general movements (pushups, or a few pull-ups, or a couple of minutes of walking on the treadmill), then a few light sets of the specific exercise I'm going to do. But nothing that will tax the body for what's to come.

With this technique, I encourage you to use a stopwatch, regular watch, or other form of timer. If your gym has a clock with an easily readable "second" hand, that's fine, too. Otherwise, you will need to count your 30 seconds of rest in your head, which is not as accurate. That 30 seconds will tend to turn into a LOT longer timespan as you go through the workout, and it's critical to keep it constant.

The timer I use has big numbers. I just set it for the TOTAL workout time. If it's 20 minutes, I set it for 20 minutes. During the workout itself, I then mentally note the time I finish the set and count the time from there. For example, if I finish a set at 16:45 on my timer, I have until 16:15 for rest.

On Day 1, start with a weight you could normally do for about six reps or so. Start your timer AFTER you finish your first set. (If you're not using a timer, note the time on the clock so you know when you're done.)

Get set on the exercise and perform ONLY three REPS with that weight, even though you CAN do about six. DO NOT go anywhere near failure on this first set. Even on successive sets, we're NOT taking any of them to absolute failure. The key here is training volume, not training to failure.

When you've done your three reps, rest 30 seconds. Then do three more reps. Rest 30 seconds. Repeat these three rep sets with those 30 seconds of rest until you are unable to get thee reps with that weight anymore. This could take anywhere from two to 10 minutes (maybe more, maybe less), depending on the exercise and amount of weight you're using.

Here's the key

If you're on rep 2 and it feels like you would have to really push to get that third rep, STOP!

The idea is NOT to push yourself to the max on each set, but to stop short of it and train based on volume. So if you're on rep 2 and you think you could get three but it would be a struggle, that's the end of the line for THAT weight. ALWAYS keep the "do or die" rep in you. THIS IS ABSOLUTELY CRITICAL.

If you're doing squats or deadlifts (which we ARE the first time through) remove 10 pounds from each side of the bar—20 pounds total. (If you started with 315, you now have 295 on the bar). Start again doing three rep sets and continue with the 30-second rest period. Drop the weight by 20 pounds total whenever you can't complete three reps during a set.

NOTE: When you're using an exercise other than squats or deadlifts, go with 10-pound total drops (five pounds off each side). You drop 20 pounds with squats and deadlifts because they allow you to use relatively MORE weight than any other exercise. When doing them, if you drop only 10 pounds off, the body won't really feel the difference and you won't be able to continue as effectively—you'll have to reduce the weight again too soon.

Be sure to stick with three reps on each set. No more, no less. Your body hits a rep-range groove and will acclimate to it very quickly. This keeps your nervous system efficient because it basically gets tuned to those three rep sets. The reason we're using three reps as the "magic" number is that it IS a magic number. It's not so many reps that you build up significant metabolic waste products. It's a low enough number that you can use a lot of weight and build strength very effectively. But it's not double or singles, which would make you do TOO much weight, leading to more rapid burnout. After much experimentation, I've found three to actually BE a magic number for this training.

Basically, your body will become a MACHINE at whatever exercise you're doing.

On the final set, when your allotted workout time is up, rest for two FULL MINUTES (Aren't I generous!) Then go back to the exercise and crank out as many reps as you can with the same weight you just ended with. You'll find that you can probably get five to eight reps on that last burnout set just because of the increased rest period.

This training uses neuromuscular specificity to teach your body the absolutely MOST efficient way to perform a single exercise. Your body will learn to fire the exact sequence of muscle fibers it needs to do the exercise most efficiently. The extreme specificity also develops the exact muscles needed to perform that exercise in the most efficient pattern. This makes the quick strength gains possible.

DO NOT use different variations of the same exercise. (For example, if you're doing bench press, don't start with incline bench and then go to flat bench.) It's important to use the EXACT SAME exercise for every single set for the whole five days of workouts for maximum adaptive response.

Do your best with the 30-second rest, too. This rest period will naturally increase when you're making weight changes, but even then try to keep it as close to 30 seconds as possible. Do your best to stick with the 30 seconds.

GOOD TIP: When doing this training with a barbell exercise, like squats or deadlifts, I like to load the bar with small plates as I load it for my starting weight. For example, if you're starting with 315 pounds on the squat, don't just throw three 45-pound plates on either side. You'll be pulling a pair of those 45s off pretty quickly and that is a pain in the butt; plus, it takes up valuable training time and energy.

Instead, put two 45-pound plates on either side, then a 25-pound plate, then two 10-pound plates. It's the same weight, but when you can no longer hit 315 pounds for three reps, all you need to do is pull a small 10-pound plate off either side. This is MUCH easier than pulling 45s off either side, then loading 35s back on. This is just as true with other exercises when you're only dropping by 10 pounds total (use five-pound plates to get to your starting weight). Believe me, you'll be dropping weight fairly quickly during the first quarter to half of each training session.

Be VERY sure to keep track of your starting and ending weights (and the length of time you were able to do each) so you know what your numbers are and can improve on them the next time you do this technique. It's always nice to chart your progress, but in this case we do it because we want to literally FORCE the issue with adaptation. By steadily increasing weight, you will force your body to get stronger.

As far as stretching goes, ONLY stretch the target muscle group AFTER the final set of the workout, NOT during the workout. We want to keep as much blood in the area as possible. Even waste products like lactic acid stimulate muscle growth, and lactic acid in particular stimulates growth hormone secretion.

When you're doing this technique with squats, start getting into position at the 20-second mark, even though you have 30 seconds of rest. It takes about 10 seconds to get into position under the bar. If you start getting into position at 30, you'll be taking 40 seconds of rest.

When you are doing this technique with deadlifts and using a mixed grip (one hand over, one hand under), it's a good idea to switch your grip on alternating sets to help keep your body balanced. For example, if you grip overhand with your left hand and underhand with the right on one set, grip overhand with your right hand and underhand with your left on the next set.

Day By Day Rundown of the 5-Day Structural Attack

In this section, I'm going to give you a day-by-day diary account of how the training will most likely go for you. I've done this 5-Day Attack a number of times and experienced similar results patterns each time. I think my experience will help you know what to expect as you go through these five days, as this training is going to be unlike any you've experienced before.

Note that I'm also going to include modifications, in case you aren't able to do five days in a row. (It's tough!)

If you do the first day and feel completely trashed on Day 2, immediately switch over to the three-day version.

Here's what the overall 5-Day Structural Attack looks like:

Day 1: 20 minutes of Compound Exercise Overload on Target Exercise

- Start with a weight you can normally get about six or seven reps with.

Day 2: 25 minutes of Compound Exercise Overload on Target Exercise

- Increase the start weight according to how you feel. It may be five, 10 or 20 pounds depending on the exercise.

Day 3: 30 minutes of Compound Exercise Overload on Target Exercise

- Increase the start weight according to how you feel. Again, it may be five, 10 or 20 pounds depending on the exercise.

Day 4: 35 minutes of Compound Exercise Overload on Target Exercise

- If you can, increase the start weight according to how you feel. It may be five, 10 or 20 pounds depending on the exercise.

Day 5: 40 minutes of Compound Exercise Overload on Target Exercise

- Start with the weight you led off with on the first day.

You'll notice that the first day of training starts with 20 minutes of Compound Exercise Overload training, increasing by five minutes each day. This gradual increase provides excellent progressive increases in strength and muscle mass. On each of the first three or four days of this five-day program, you should strive to increase the weight you're using when you start.

It is absolutely ESSENTIAL that you EAT A LOT on these five training days. You're going to be burning a TON of calories, and you'll need to fuel your body and the recovery process. Eat a lot of protein and plenty of carbs, and don't be shy about eating fat as well. Fat is concentrated calories, and your body is going to use them. I'm not saying eat crap food, but don't be afraid to eat fat.

Believe me, with the training you'll be doing this week, there's not much you can eat that will make you fat.

Another ESSENTIAL point: Drink a LOT of water every day. This is not an option. If you want to really maximize your results, you need to stay well-hydrated. Muscle growth happens when nutrients are available and the muscle cells are well-hydrated. By almost overflowing yourself with water, you ensure that the muscles are fully hydrated and able to maximize muscle growth.

Here's the bottom line: You are not going to gain seven pounds in a week without MOST of that being water associated with muscle. (The weight of a muscle is actually mostly water.) By drinking a lot, you ensure that you'll be able to build the most muscle possible.

On the following week (Stretch-Pause Training), DO NOT use the same exercise you used for the 5-Day Attack. Use other exercises, but don't repeat that same exercise until the second week of that training. Your body will still be trying to recover from the 5-Day Attack, and the movement pattern will be pretty well overtrained. Stay away from it and focus on other exercises. When you go back to it, you will be a LOT stronger with it!

My Deadlift Experience

Day 1: 20 minutes

Bodyweight 202 pounds

Started with 365 pounds for 4 minutes

Ended at 275 lbs for 4 minutes

Being the first day of the program and the shortest workout, this didn't feel too bad at all. After the first four or five sets, I could really feel myself getting in the groove of the exercise and developing some good efficiency. After four minutes at 365 pounds, I dropped the weight to the next level and continued. Because this was the first day, and it was a total shock to my body, I had to drop all the way down to 275 pounds, ending up there for the last four minutes. Legs felt good, but my lower back was protesting a bit toward the end.

It is CRITICAL to note here that you MUST keep strict form on every rep of every set of this training program (not that you shouldn't anyway, but it's especially important here). Because the volume is so high, any small errors will be magnified. If your form isn't perfect, reduce the weight. No exceptions.

If ever in the course of these sessions, you find yourself REALLY suffering—you're compromising your form even when you reduce the weight—stop your timer and take a minute or two of rest. You're not letting the workout time run down while you're taking the break; you're just pausing the workout. Stretch out a bit to get things feeling better. Restart the timer, then get back into it. But don't give up! It probably won't come to that on the FIRST day, but it may as you go through on the next few days.

Day 2: 25 minutes

Bodyweight 204 pounds

Started with 385 pounds for 6-1/2 minutes: 20-pound increase over Day 1

Ended at 325 pounds for 10 minutes

Today, I added 20 pounds to the exercise. This is important: You should try to add to your starting weight for at least the first three and, hopefully, four sessions this week. I felt stronger and was able to keep going with that heavier weight for longer than I could with a lighter weight yesterday.

When deadlifting, I find it best to hold the breath for at least the bottom half to two-thirds of the movement. This helps increase spinal and core stability by keeping everything still. When you pass that halfway mark on the way up, THEN start breathing out, basically pushing breath out through pursed lips, like you're blowing up a balloon. On the way down, it's just as critical. Breathe in at the top. Then, when you hit the halfway point, hold your breath to increase core solidity. This helps protect your lower back.

Overall, the 25 minutes of training still didn't feel too bad today. Tough, but not too bad.

Day 3: 30 minutes

Bodyweight 206 pounds

Started with 405 pounds for 3 minutes: 20-pound increase over Day 2

Ended at 285 pounds for 10 minutes

I felt like I couldn't eat enough food even though I was eating a LOT. I could feel my metabolism roaring. Even with the air-conditioning on in the house, I felt like I was roasting. This training is VERY effective for building mass. I felt I was getting bigger even in just the first three days.

This was a tougher workout for sure. Since I'm feeling stronger, I was able to again start at a higher weight and stay at a higher weight, at least for a while. As I kept going, I ended up dropping down to 285 pounds which, while less than yesterday, was still more than I ended up at on the first day. That's great!

Remember, this week you shouldn't be doing anything but this training if you can help it (in terms of physical activity, at least). It's extremely hard on the body, and it won't take much to push your recovery systems over the edge. So NO cardio and, if at all possible, no manual labor.

Day 4: 35 minutes

Bodyweight 207 pounds

Started with 425 pounds for 4-1/2 minutes: 20-pound increase over Day 3

Ended at 225 pounds for 5 minutes

Remember when I mentioned that you can stop the timer and take a break for a couple of minutes before continuing? I had to do this a couple of times in this session. My lower back, while not exhausted, was so choked with blood that it was starting to affect my form. So I stopped the timer, walked around a bit, stretched out a bit, hung from the chin-up bars, and sat down a little. When the blood and waste products had been cleared (it took about two minutes), I started back in and got the timer going again.

This was a particularly tough day. I can tell I'm really getting close to the wall. Just where I like to be! I was able to again start at a heavier weight (a total of 60 pounds heavier than I started with!). But I had to start dropping weight a lot faster.

After the initial 4-1/2 minutes at 425 pounds, I had to drop weight three more times in the next five minutes.

One of the things I found VERY helpful when doing deadlifting here was to go over to the dip stand and hold the lockout position, just letting my legs hang (relax the midsection completely and dangle the legs) to get traction on the spine and spinal erector muscles. With the deadlift, the area gets so congested with blood, it can affect the short-term recovery. By taking a couple of minutes to allow some circulation, I was able to get back into the exercise without much problem. Until it got pumped up again, of course. Then I had to take another short break.

I've also found it helpful to sit on a bench with my hands on the bench beside me and just take tension off the lower back so it doesn't have to hold up my upper body. This helps get some circulation through to flush out waste products.

Day 5: 40 minutes

Bodyweight 209 pounds

Started with 365 pounds for 7 minutes: Back to Day 1 start weight

Ended at 245 pounds for 22 minutes

Today's workout was tough right from the start, even to get up the motivation to go to the gym and do it! At this point, your body is very much on the way to overtraining, which is the goal. This final workout will really seal the deal. But the cool thing is, I've gained about seven pounds of bodyweight this week! At 40 minutes of workout time, the clock is not your friend today. This is the toughest one to get through of the whole week. You'll really find out what you're made of.

Even after five days of doing the same exercise over and over for a TON of sets, I'm still able to go longer (almost twice as long) with the same weight as I did on the first day. This no doubt goes contrary to everything you've read about how muscles recover. Technically, the amount of weight you can lift should DROP every day, not go UP every day.

Today, I used 30-pound weight drops instead of 20. On this last day, because your body is at the end of the line, the larger weight drops may be necessary to allow you to keep going for a decent amount of time on each new weight. If you drop only 20, you'll be dropping again within a couple of sets, and that takes up time.

If you're using an exercise other than deadlifts or squats, you can drop the weight by 20 pounds instead of the usual 10.

Be sure to eat a LOT every single one of these training days. This is absolutely critical to getting the most out of this week. You need to fuel up your body to maximize results. It will pay off in gains, I promise. And because your metabolism is roaring trying to keep up, you will hardly gain any fat.

On the very last set, after taking the two minutes of rest at the end of 40 minutes, I decided to go for broke and really see how many reps I could do with my end weight of 245 pounds.

Turns out that number was 20! Believe me, that was a TOUGH 20 reps after 40 minutes of deadlifting. I'm happy to be done with this week. But at same time, I'm looking forward to doing it again in the near future! This was some of THE most effective mass building I've EVER done.

Side note: Bodyweight of 213 on Sunday (2 days later). That's 11 pounds in one week!

Modifications to the 5-Day Structural Attack

This is, quite honestly, one of the toughest five days you'll ever come across in your training, especially when you use squats or deadlifts. Here are a couple of modifications you can make to this 5-Day Attack to help increase the chances you'll finish it.

1. Change the 5-Day Attack to a 3-Day Attack

If you are an intermediate trainer, consider a 3-Day Attack instead. Here's what it looks like:

> *Day 1: 20 minutes of target exercise*
>
> *Day 2: off (instead of 25 minutes of target exercise)*
>
> *Day 3: 25 minutes of target exercise*
>
> *Day 4: off (instead of 35 minutes of target exercise)*
>
> *Day 5: 30 minutes of target exercise*

Even with this modification, it will be VERY tough and VERY effective. You won't be hitting the muscles every day, but you will still get a great emergency response from the body.

2. Take Rest Periods WITHIN the Training Sessions

If you find, as you're going through the training, that you have to stop and rest longer than 20 or 30 seconds, that's completely fine! I've done that myself. When you find you have to reduce weights too quickly, or if lactic acid is making the exercises unbearable to do (it happens), stop the timer and take a couple of minutes or more of complete rest (no changing weights). Then reset the timer when you begin again. See how that helps you to recover.

The key thing is to stop and restart the timer so you aren't taking up training time with your rest. This should allow you to keep going. Do it whenever you feel you have to.

Stretch-Pause Training

The final two weeks of the Muscle Explosion Program is Stretch-Pause Training. If the name sounds a lot like Rest-Pause Training, it's because it IS a lot like Rest-Pause Training. But it has a couple of CRITICAL differences that, in my experience, make it even MORE effective than traditional Rest-Pause Training (which, by the way, is VERY effective). If you're familiar with DC Training, you might recognize some of the general principles at work here. (DC Training is based primarily on a version of Rest-Pause Training.)

I'll start with a quick explanation of what Rest-Pause Training is. It's simple. You do a full set until you can't perform any more reps. Generally, you want to aim for eight to 10 reps on the first part. Then you take a brief rest, normally 10 to 20 seconds.

Then you repeat the same exercise with the same weight for as many MORE reps as you can. You can then either stop or, after another brief rest, do as many MORE reps as you can again.

What this allows you to do is get more reps with weight you could normally only get eight to 10 reps for. It works so well because it increases the overall workload on the muscles at the most effective point in the set—near momentary muscular failure. You're basically taking the muscles to failure three times in a very short space of time.

This is VERY effective for building muscle, and I considered adding it as-is into this phase of the program. But then I came up with a BETTER way to do Rest-Pause Training.

I call it Stretch-Pause Training. Here's how it's different:

Like regular Rest-Pause Training, you start with a weight you could normally get eight to 10 reps for (aim for the 10-rep mark). It's important to keep strict form and concentrate on keeping tension on the target muscles. No bouncing, cheating, or momentum here. Complete your full set of 10 reps. If you can get more, do more; we want to get to failure here.

Rest 20 seconds.

Now, instead of doing the SAME exercise again, we're going to take a page out of the Tissue Remodeling Training technique and go to a stretch-accentuated exercise. But instead of doing partial reps in just the stretch position, we're going to do FULL-range reps with a FOCUS on the stretch.

You are going to HOLD that stretch position at the bottom of EVERY REP for at least three to five seconds (count to five at the bottom—that will work just fine). You'll aim for six to eight reps.

Get a STRONG stretch on every rep. It's not pleasant, but this stretches out the fascia, giving the muscles room to grow.

When you are done with that set, rest 20 seconds. Then go back to the FIRST exercise. You're going to use the SAME weight, but you're going to try to get as many more reps as you can. HOWEVER, you're going to work only the top, partial range of motion of the exercise—for example, the top one-third of bench press.

When doing this final portion of the Stretch-Pause set, use a VERY DELIBERATE movement, pausing at the top and bottom of each partial rep for at least a full second. This will keep momentum out of the exercise and allow you to focus on maximizing the tension on the target muscle group. Squeeze the muscles HARD and really get your mind into the muscle. You want to develop as much tension as you can in the target muscles to maximize the overall effect of the Stretch-Pause set.

Basically, it looks like this: full-range exercise -> rest 20 seconds -> stretch exercise -> rest 20 seconds -> partial/ top-range exercise.

When you are using this technique with squats and deadlifts, don't do a stretch-accentuated exercise in the middle. There aren't any stretch exercises that will be more effective for building mass than simply doing another set of squats or deadlifts here. That being said, you STILL want to do partial/top-range movement in the third part of the set. Here's what it would look like for squats and deadlifts:

Full-range squats or deadlifts -> rest 20 seconds -> full-range squats or deadlifts -> rest 20 seconds -> partial/ top-range squats or deadlifts.

If you find you can't get a good stretch on any shoulder exercises, you can follow this outline with shoulder presses, too. Shoulders can be tough to get a good stretch on, but the technique is still very effective using any form of shoulder press.

Why Does It Work?

Stretch-Pause Training is effective because it helps stretch out the fascia (the connective tissue "pillowcases" surrounding your muscles), giving the muscles more room to grow. I go into greater detail on this in the Tissue Remodeling Training section. Basically, stretching the muscles while they're pumped full of blood helps to "wiggle" the fascia and expand it a bit. With this expansion of the "pillowcase" around them, the muscles have space to expand into. Normally, when you do Rest-Pause Training, you're only able to do one or two reps with your working weight. But when you do PARTIAL range of motion in the strongest part of the exercise ONLY, you can immediately get more reps with that weight and increase the time under tension of the muscles. More tension means more muscle growth.

Don't be surprised if you feel like your muscles are about to rip right out of your skin at this point. The stretch-position exercise also helps to recruit and activate more muscle fibers. When you go to the fully contracted position with heavy weight and greater tension, you are hitting almost ALL available muscle fibers.

It's a POWERFUL technique and, believe me, you don't need many sets to blow your muscles up FAST.

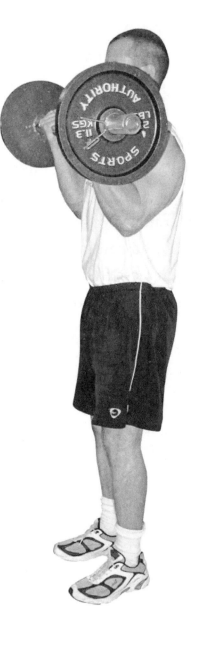
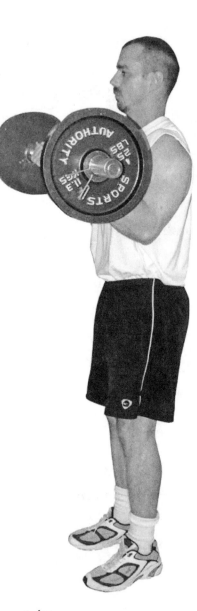

Stretch-pause training 1/3 top range
BARBELL CURLS

The Core Combo

The Core Combo is very simple. It includes components designed to improve your abdominal and lower back strength, as well as the rotator cuff to keep your shoulders strong and healthy. These areas are CRITICAL for assisting with overall muscle development.

This combination is done to ensure that no muscles are underdeveloped. Generally, if a person does not do regular deadlifting or other direct lower back work, the lower back can easily become a weak link. This may lead to lower back pain and decrease the weight you can lift with exercises such as squats.

With this program, however, deadlifts and stiff-legged deadlifts are key exercises, so that is not a major issue. The lower back gets a good amount of work, which is why I've included only light lower back work like hyperextensions in the Core Combo.

The Core Combo is done after almost every single workout (the exact times you will use the combo are listed in the program phases in the Appendix). The abdominal work will be targeted toward increasing overall core and ab strength rather than how your abs look (meaning, you're not going to be doing a lot of crunching type movements but exercises that target core stability).

Working the rotator cuff is VERY important in a strength and mass program. The four muscles of the rotator cuff (infraspinatus, supraspinatus, subscapularis, and teres minor) serve to stabilize the humerus (your upper arm bone) in the shoulder joint. When you do heavy bench pressing and shoulder pressing, rotator cuff strength is ESSENTIAL for keeping your shoulders healthy.

In real-world terms, working the cuff regularly can result in improvements of up to 20 pounds in a week in your bench press strength! I've included regular cuff work to protect your shoulders and improve your upper body pressing strength.

The Core Combo should take no more than five minutes or so to complete. You go from abs straight to lower back, straight to rotator cuff with minimal rest between sets (about 20 to 30 seconds).

Ab Exercises

Use any of the three ab exercises listed on the next few pages, or feel free to use your own. (Remember, I've chosen exercises targeted for core strength.) The number of sets is limited, so work them hard and make them count! Aim for six to 10 reps per set and go to failure. Rest about 30 seconds between ab sets. I would recommend using only one exercise in your ab sets to make setup easier.

To develop core strength that is useful in heavy training, the abs need to be pushed hard with good resistance, not with endless reps with very little weight. Don't be shy about pushing yourself hard when it comes to adding resistance to the exercises.

Lower Back Exercises

For the lower back, use an isolation exercise such as the regular hyperextension, the hyper crunch, or the reverse hyperextension. Since you'll be doing regular heavy deadlifting and stiff-legged deadlifts, the lower back will get plenty of heavy work.

You can do lower back work for higher reps with just bodyweight or add resistance (by holding a dumbbell or barbell plate), then use lower reps to build strength in the area. Rest 30 seconds between sets.

Rotator Cuff Exercises

The rotator cuff muscles are essential for keeping the shoulder joint strong and healthy. Working them regularly is important. I've included an exercise I call the Three-In-One Rotator Cuff Exercise. It combines several different cuff movements into one movement. It's effective and saves time while giving your rotator cuff a complete workout.

Do one arm at a time, and take no rest between sets for each arm, basically going back and forth between right and left arm. Do sets of 10 to 12 reps per arm and don't push this muscle group to failure. The idea is to strengthen but not exhaust. You don't need heavy weight for this exercise.

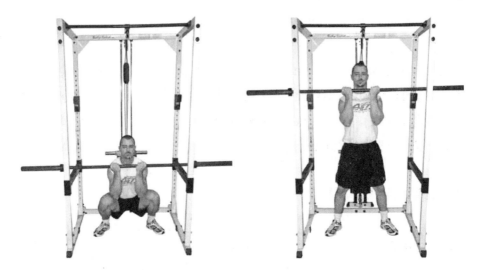

BARBELL CURL SQUATS

Curl Squat

Why Is This Exercise So Effective?

This is an extraordinary exercise for building supporting strength and stability in the core muscles, especially for movements such as squats and deadlifts.

This exercise is simple to do with dumbbells, barbell, or cables. Each has its strengths and drawbacks, of course. The movement is similar to the front squat without any of the support you would normally get from your shoulders. All the support tension goes onto your abs!

The Barbell Version

Set the squat rack up so that the racks are one notch below where you would normally set them for squats. You do this because by the time you're done, it may be very hard to get the bar back to where you normally rack it. Set the safety rails just above where you normally set them for regular squats the first time you try this, too. When you develop a better feel for how it's done, you can lower them a little to get a fuller range of motion.

Step in front of the bar and hold it in the top position of the barbell curl. Now stand up, unracking the bar. Don't allow your elbows to brace against your midsection. This takes away from the supporting tension on the abs. Take a step back and get your feet set. Now, holding the bar in that top curl position through the entire movement, squat down as far as you can, then come back up. You don't actually curl the bar while doing the squat, you just hold it in the top curl position.

Hold your breath during the majority of this movement to keep greater stability in your core. Start holding as you start to go below the halfway point, and continue to hold it until you're about halfway back up. If you don't want to or are unable to hold your breath, exhale through pursed lips (as though you're blowing up a balloon). Keeping the breath held will maximize core stability and allow your abs to function more effectively during the movement. Since this exercise uses relatively light weight compared to a regular squat, holding your breath is not nearly as potentially dangerous. If you do feel lightheaded, rack the bar and rest.

Holding the resistance in front of your body, as you do in this exercise, takes away the shoulder support you would normally get with a front squat. The required supporting tension goes directly on the core muscles, which have to contract hard throughout the entire movement to keep the barbell from falling forward.

This exercise helps you get a feel for using the abs during a squat, which is extremely important for maximizing your squat strength. Using the abs while squatting does not come naturally and is very rarely taught or explained. But this exercise helps to greatly strengthen the abs for that specific purpose, making this a very powerful core and overall strength-building exercise.

When doing the exercise for the first time, start with just the bar, no matter how strong you are. This will help you get a feel for the movement, where to set the safety rails, and how far down you can comfortably go. When you're comfortable, work your way up slowly from there, as fatigue will come quickly. It's a movement your body will be totally unused to, no matter how many abdominal exercises you've done in your training career. The core muscles will tire before your legs do. Be sure to keep your lower back arched and tight while performing this movement.

If you are able to, go all the way down until your elbows touch your knees. This will give you the fullest range of motion. Tense the abs hard, especially at the bottom as you are coming back up. For extra resistance, pause at the bottom for a few seconds. This will give you the best feel for how the abs should be used when squatting.

With this exercise, holding the resistance in front of the body (like in a front squat) allows you to keep a more vertical body position. The tension will go onto the abs, but be aware that there will also be some tension to the lower back. Because you are holding the weight out in front of you, the lower back must also contract to help stabilize the spine. As you keep up with the exercise, your lower back will get stronger.

Another great benefit is that your breathing muscles (the intercostals) never get a chance to relax during this movement. From top to bottom and back up (even while you're "resting" at the top), your breathing muscles are being challenged by the weight they are being forced to support. This can build up great lung capacity and breathing strength (excellent for athletes who need great cardio capacity). And it carries directly over to your work capacity in the regular barbell squat.

The Cable Version

The cable version is essentially the same in form as the barbell version but with one big difference: The angle of the cable adds forward pulling resistance. This adds another tension to the abs because, in addition to supporting the weight, they're also forced to contract to keep you from falling forward. The exercise doesn't require as much stability control as the barbell version, however, and your breathing muscles won't be challenged as much.

Get the bar to the top of the curl position, take a step back, then perform the exercise as you would with the barbell.

If you have an adjustable-height cable setup, it's best to start this exercise with the pulley set a few notches up. (This makes it easier to get into the start position.) If you just have a low-pulley, you'll need to curl the weight up into position to start the movement.

The Dumbbell Version

The dumbbell version can be done two ways: with two dumbbells or with one. The execution with two dumbbells is exactly the same as with the barbell version, the only difference being that you have to curl or clean the weight up to the top of the curl position to do the exercise.

If you are using only one dumbbell, this one-sided tension will allow you to put torque on the abs to work the sides (switch sides with each set for a balanced workout). When you are using one dumbbell, you can also drop your elbow inside your knees to go down deeper. You can get your butt right down by your heels with this one. Very challenging!

Common Errors

1. **Doing this exercise after a bicep workout**

    As you can imagine, performing this exercise is not going be as effective if you've just finished a bicep workout. The biceps will already be fatigued, and you'll limit the amount of weight you can use and how long you can hold it. Use this exercise on non-bicep training days.

2. **Going too fast**

    Dropping down quickly in the squat will put extra stress on the biceps as you come up and reduce the tension on the abs. This exercise should be done very deliberately, with no bouncing or fast movements. If you have a tendency to do either, pause at the bottom for a few seconds to stop the bouncing.

3. **Using too much weight**

    Since the legs are so much stronger, it's tempting to use too much weight for this exercise. Remember, our goal here is NOT to work the legs or the biceps, but to work the abs. The legs and the biceps are only here to help push the abs. If your biceps fatigue before your abs get a good workout, you need to reduce the weight.

4. **Leaning forward**

   Try to keep your upper body as vertical as possible. It's very similar to a front squat. Having the weight in front of you allows you to stay vertical more easily. Leaning forward will cause the barbell to shift forward, which will put more tension on the biceps, causing them to fatigue prematurely. As you start to fatigue, you will notice you have a tendency to lean forward. This is because the supporting abs are weakening. Do your best to keep vertical. Once you start to move too far forward, end the set.

5. **Bar too close to collarbones**

   If the bar gets too close to the collarbones, you will lose some of the tension in the abs. Keep the bar at least a few inches away to maximize the supporting tension and torque demanded of the abs. If it comes too close, you may be tempted to rest the bar on your collarbones, which will turn it into an uncomfortable front squat.

6. **Letting the elbows brace strongly against the midsection**

   If you let the elbows press strongly into the midsection, you take away some of the tension on the abs. A little contact is fine, especially as you tire, but don't rely on using this technique or you make the exercise less effective. Letting the elbows sink in will also tend to hunch your back over, putting pressure on the lower back. This will pull your torso and center of balance forward, putting more tension on the biceps, making you dig the elbows in more! Keep the elbows out front, away from your body, and you'll keep a better body position and do a more effective set.

Tricks

1. **Look forward and slightly up**

   When you squat, keep looking forward and slightly up. This will help you keep an arch in your lower back and keep you from leaning forward. You want to avoid forward lean, as it causes the biceps to fatigue prematurely.

2. **Don't breathe too deeply in or out as you are coming down or pushing back up**

   Breathing too much during this exercise reduces core stability and can compromise form. For best core stabilization, keep your breath carefully controlled. At the bottom, you can hold your breath for a few moments to get the most solid stability. As you come up, exhale through pursed lips after you've come about one-quarter to one-half of the way. This technique shouldn't be used if you have blood pressure issues, however, as it does cause an increase in blood pressure.

Keep a careful eye on how you feel if you do choose to do this. If you feel any dizziness, end the set and don't use this technique the next set.

3. **Pause at the bottom**

   To really maximize the tension on the abs, pause for a few seconds at the bottom and focus on really squeezing and tightening your abs hard. As you start to come back up, try to push with your abs as well. This will help you feel what it's like to use the abs to help push out of the bottom when doing regular barbell squats.

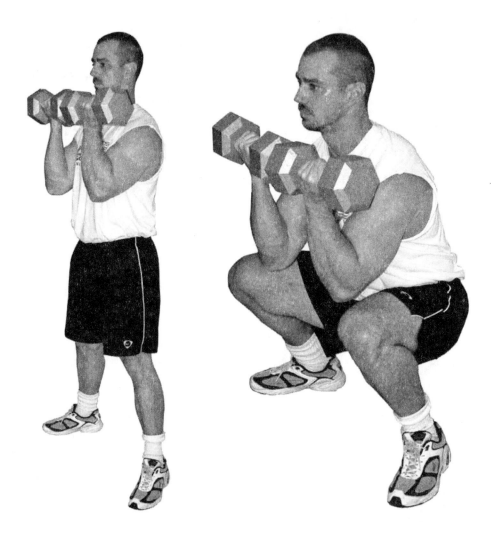

DUMBBELL CURL SQUATS

Two-Dumbbell Ball Twist

Why Is This Exercise So Effective?

Using only a Swiss Ball and two dumbbells, you can achieve an extraordinary ab-tightening contraction around the entire midsection musculature. This exercise places great stretch, along with great tension, on the obliques, forcing quick abdominal development.

How to Do It

You need two dumbbells and a Swiss Ball (I tell you how to do this on a regular flat bench in the Tricks section below). A smaller-size ball is better for this exercise, though any ball will work.

Lie on your back with your knees bent and your feet fairly wide apart. You need a good base of support so you don't roll off to the side of the ball. Hold two equal-weight dumbbells at arms-length directly above you. Press them together while doing this exercise (if they're separated, they'll move around more, making the exercise less efficient). Start with fairly light dumbbells the first time you try this movement.

Keeping your head facing directly up/forwards and your hips horizontal, lower both dumbbells slowly and under complete control down to the left. Hold your breath and tighten your midsection as you come down to the fully twisted position. Prepare to push hard against the ground with your left foot to maintain your balance.

Your left arm is going to bend to about 90 degrees at the elbow as you lower the dumbbells to the side while your right arm should stay perfectly straight. Your upper body should stay in the same position on the ball—no rolling to the opposite side to compensate for the weight to the side. This torque is what makes the exercise so valuable. Bending your lower arm is critical to keeping your torso in the same position on the ball.

Because you are using two separate dumbbells, you create a very different stress on the abdominal area than any you've experienced before.

When you're at the bottom, your upper left arm will touch the surface of the ball. (Don't let it rest or lose tension at this point!) Reverse the direction by simultaneously pulling with your right side abs and pushing with your left side abs. The right arm movement is similar to a rear delt lateral, while the left arm movement is similar to a dumbbell press.

Remember to keep the dumbbells pressed together tightly. The opposing tension in the abs puts a lot of torque across the whole area. Be very sure you're not just pushing with the bottom arm but also pulling with the top arm.

Be sure not to bounce out of the bottom. Try to feel a stretch in the right side as you start the change of direction.

If you have any lower back pain issues, this exercise does put some stress on the lower back. If you do try it, go very light and take it very slowly.

Common Errors

1. **Separating the dumbbells**
   Keep them pressed together throughout the movement. If they separate, they're harder to control, and you disperse the tension on the abs.

2. **Rolling around on the ball**
   For best results, be sure to keep yourself as stationary as possible on the ball. If you roll to the side, you take some of the torque off the abs and lose effectiveness.

3. **Moving too quickly**
   This is NOT a ballistic exercise. There should be no bouncing or fast movements involved. Lower the dumbbells slowly to the sides and change direction very deliberately by using muscle power, not bouncing.

Tricks

1. Change the arc

You can bring the dumbbells down at various angles to the torso to change where the exercise hits your abs. By bringing it down beside your head, you'll hit the upper area of your obliques. By bringing it down toward your hip, you'll hit the lower area. Just remember to always keep your head looking straight up and set your feet wide apart for the best base of support.

2. Use a flat bench instead

You can also do this exercise on a flat bench. Instead of lying flat on the bench as you normally would for a bench press, you'll be resting only your upper back on the end of the bench.

To get into this position, sit on the very end of the bench. Now move your butt off the bench and squat down in front of it. Lean back and place your upper back on the bench end. Keep your hips down and set your feet fairly wide apart.

This is the position you should maintain while doing the exercise. The bench is a more solid surface, and it is just as effective for the exercise. But there won't be any surface to make contact with the bottom arm as you lower the weight down. Keep an eye on how far down you go to the side. All other techniques still apply.

3. Use a heavier weight

If you are using a heavy weight, you will need to shift your upper body somewhat to the other side of the ball in order to stay on the ball. The increased resistance will make up for it.

Be extra careful that the dumbbells don't separate. It is much harder to control heavier dumbbells if they do.

As you rotate back up, exhale through pursed lips to keep stability in your abs and so you don't pass out.

Push VERY hard with the same side leg as the weight is on. You'll need all the help you can get.

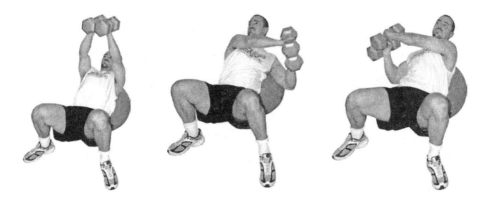

TWO DUMBBELL BALL TWISTS

Abdominal Sit-Up

Why Is This Exercise So Effective?

This is a sit-up movement that works the abs instead of the hip flexors. It will work all the muscles in your midsection in one exercise.

The standard crunch only addresses part of the function of the abdominals. This exercise targets the flexed (arched back) range of motion of the abs and uses the weight of your entire torso as resistance.

Lie on your back on the floor. Roll up a towel or mat and slip it beneath your lower back just above the waistband. (The size of the towel affects your body position during this movement; use a fairly large towel.).

Your knees should be bent about 90 degrees. Keep your feet close together and your knees fairly wide apart. This prevents the hip flexors from having a direct line of pull, minimizing their involvement. Do not anchor your feet or have someone hold them down. This automatically activates the hip flexors. You will get the most out of this exercise by minimizing their involvement.

The difficulty of this exercise depends on where you hold your hands. The hardest position is above your head at arms-length, then beside your head, then across your chest, then straight down between your legs or at your sides. Start with the easiest position first. Progress to the other positions as you get stronger.

You are now ready to crunch.

Keeping your torso straight and stiff, start the sit-up by tightening your lower abs. As you continue up, imagine trying to push your face up against the ceiling (think up, not around). When you reach about 25 to 30 degrees above horizontal, hold for a second and squeeze hard.

Keep your back in contact with the towel at all times and always maintain tension in the abs. Lower yourself down slowly and under control. Do not just drop back to the ground. The negative portion of this exercise is extremely effective.

Common Errors

1. **Using momentum**

   Do not swing yourself up to get started. Always squeeze yourself up using ab power. Start with the easiest positions first, for example, arms down at your sides. If you are having trouble doing this exercise, try using a slant board (with your head higher up).

2. **Losing tension at the top**

   This occurs when you come too far up. Always maintain contact with the towel and keep tension in your abs.

3. **Allowing the glutes to come off the ground**

   Keep the glutes on the ground at all times. The glutes tend to come up at the start of the rep, when your abs are first trying to get your body off the ground and your back is pivoting over the towel.

4. **Coming up too far**

   This error actually takes tension off the abs just when they should be getting the most tension. Keep your lower back in contact with the towel throughout the exercise.

5. **Improper towel placement**

   The towel should be just above the waistband area in the small of the back. Placing it too high or too low will affect the exercise negatively.

Tricks

1. **Move your hand position through the set**

   When you get stronger at this exercise, start with your hands over your head. When you fail with that, continue with your hands beside your head, then continue with

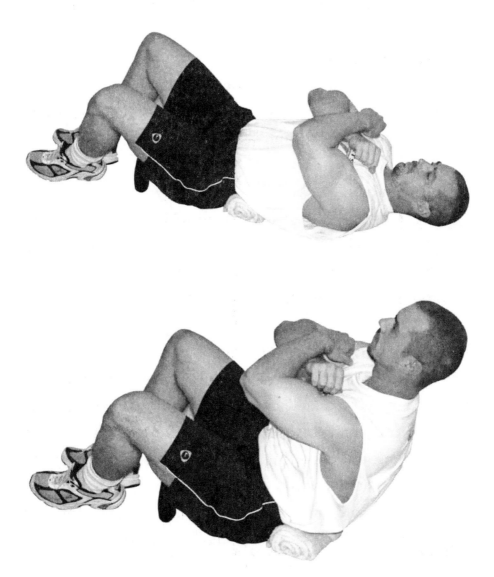

Abdominal Sit-Ups

hands across the chest, then hands at your sides or between your legs to finish. It is a merciless drop set.

2. **Use extra resistance**

   Hold a weight plate in your hands. Start very light, say five to 10 pounds, as balance can be a problem, especially because your feet should not be anchored.

3. **Spot yourself**

   Extra resistance, as described above, can also be used to spot yourself. Hold the weight plate out in front of you instead of behind you. This will act as a counterbalance and help pull your body up.

4. **Use an extra hard contraction**

   This technique will give you an extra hard contraction: Once you come up to about 25 degrees, bring your arms in so your forearms are in front of your face (like a boxer covering up). Pivoting just below the rib cage using your upper abs only, crunch your elbows down toward your hips and squeeze hard, exhaling completely. Your lower abs will not move at all. This makes it look like a two-part movement: the sit-up, then stop, then the crunch over.

   You can also give yourself a little spot by grabbing onto your legs and pulling over.

5. **Work the sides**

   To work the sides more during this movement, come up to 25 degrees. Then do a twisting crunch over to the side. Don't do the twist as you are coming up in the sit-up. Do it after you are up to about 25 degrees.

6. **Breathe at the top**

   Try holding the contraction at the top and breathing in and out a few times. This will really force your abs to contract.

7. **Lengthwise on a bench**

   Lie lengthwise along a bench with the towel under your lower back. Your shoulders should be just off the end of the bench so you can stretch back and down a little. The edge of the bench should be just below the shoulder blades. Your head and arms will be hanging off the end of the bench. This will give you a greater range of motion. Execute the movement the same way.

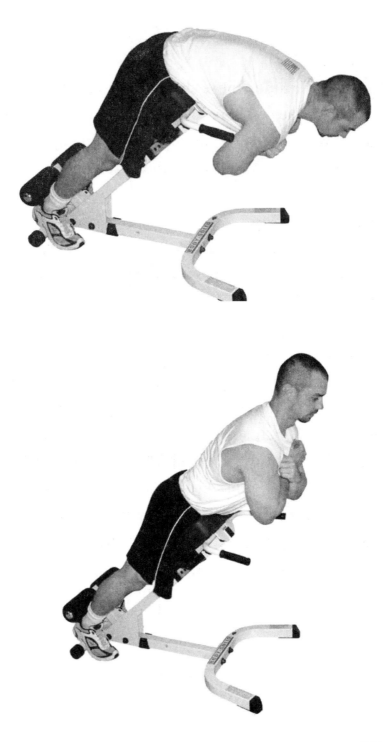

HYPER CRUNCH

Hyper Crunch

Why Is This Exercise So Effective?

This variation of the hyperextension is far more effective than the typical hyperextension for training the spinal erectors directly. The secret is not bending at the hips but flexing the spine at the vertebrae themselves.

It is better to have a rounded pad for this version. If you don't and the exercise is too uncomfortable, fold a mat and put it on top of the thigh pads.

Instead of resting your thighs on the pads, rest your midsection on the pads. The edge of the pad should be just under your rib cage rather than at the hips.

Suck in your gut for comfort. This is especially important on the way down. If you have a potbelly, this exercise may be uncomfortable. This exercise is NOT recommended if you are pregnant as you will not be able to position yourself on the bench safely. Stick to the regular hyperextension.

Crunch over the edge of the pad, rounding your lower back until your head is down. You can hold your hands crossed in front of your chest if you like.

Crunch back up using only the spinal erectors. This exercise uses only spinal flexion and extension, not hip flexion and extension, removing the glutes as a prime mover and using them only isometrically. Squeeze hard at the top and repeat.

The downside to this movement is that it can feel uncomfortable on the abdomen. It should not be done by those with large bellies. To ease pressure on the abdomen, inhale and exhale only at the top of the movement and suck in your gut during the movement.

Common Errors

1. **Not curling the abdomen over the bench**
   The major advantage of this exercise lies in curling the abdomen, i.e., flexing the spine, over the edge of the bench. If you don't flex the spine, you won't fully work the erector spinae muscles through their full range of motion.

2. **Using momentum**
   Never use momentum on any lower back exercise. This can be very dangerous as it places stress on the spine when it's in a vulnerable position.

Tricks

1. **Imagine extending one vertebra at a time as you come up**
    This imagery will help you activate the spinal erectors. When you visualize each one extending in a sequence, each of the small spinal erector muscles will fire in order. You can also visualize yourself curling your back around a ball to achieve the same effect.

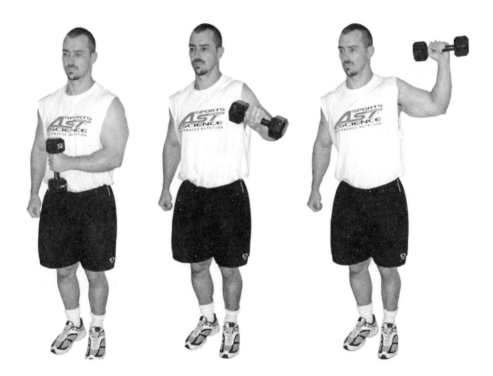

3 IN 1 ROTATOR CUFF RAISES

Three-In-One Rotator Cuff Raise

Why Is This Exercise So Effective?

Maintaining a strong rotator cuff muscle group is essential for optimum shoulder stability and strength. This exercise combines aspects of three different rotator cuff exercises, improving your efficiency when you exercise your rotator cuff muscles.

Start in a standing position with your upper arm vertical, your forearm crossed in front horizontally, and your shoulder internally rotated.

Hold the dumbbell in front of your abdomen. This is similar to the start position of what is called the Lying "L" Raise (a common rotator cuff exercise), where you lie on your side on a bench. In this exercise, though, you are in a standing position.

During this entire movement, keep a constant 90 degree bend in your elbow.

Externally rotate and abduct your shoulder (raise your upper arm up and to the side while bringing the dumbbell up and back).

While you raise your upper arm to a horizontal position, raise your forearm to a vertical position.

This should be accomplished in a smooth motion.

This is a much more time-efficient method of working the rotator cuff, as you hit three basic types of rotator cuff movements in one movement.

Common Errors

1. **Throwing the weights up**

   Don't use momentum on this exercise. You will get far more out of it if you strive for slow, controlled movements, focusing on continuous tension. Throwing the weight up is just going through the motions. You might also injure the sensitive structures of the rotator cuff.

2. **Improper timing on the movement**

   The movement should be a smooth, balanced transition from one position to the other. Choppy or jerky timing will reduce effectiveness.

3. **Moving your upper body excessively**

   If you find your torso bobbing forward and backward to get the weight up, you are using too much weight.

This exercise is most useful when done with strict form and continuous tension. Be sure you aren't trying to heave the dumbbells.

Tricks

1. **Change where you start and finish the exercise**

   You can try an alternate starting position that will keep more tension on the shoulders. Instead of holding your forearms horizontal and the dumbbells directly in front of your abdomen, try to keep your forearms up and the dumbbells held just under your chin.

   You will almost look like a boxer in the guard position. The position also resembles the top position of a two-dumbbell hammer curl if you finish with the dumbbells just under your chin. When you start the movement, let the dumbbells dip down slightly before you swing them around and start the rotator cuff movement.

NUTRITION

In muscle and strength building, training is a HUGE part of your success. But nutrition is the other HUGE part of the equation. Without good nutrition, all the hard work at the gym won't get you far. If you have been training awhile and read some, you probably have a decent background in nutrition and a fairly good idea of what to eat.

I'm going to depart from the standard "meal plan" approach and simply lay out the overall nutrition strategies we use in this program. You can select the foods you want to eat and how much to eat in the context of the program (with some guidance, of course).

With the Muscle Explosion Program, I take a VERY different approach to nutrition. I start your muscle-building adventure with a strict diet.

Bear with me as I explain the reasoning. THEN you'll see the real power of this approach.

The Slingshot Effect

Think back to the last time you were on a fat-loss diet. You weren't eating all that much in an effort to get that caloric deficit to achieve fat loss. As you kept up with the reduced-calorie eating, your body adapted by becoming more efficient with the food you were putting in. Now remember what happened when you came OFF of that diet.

You immediately increased bodyweight and probably muscle mass as well. With the increased food intake, your body immediately cranked up your metabolism and started storing all the nutrients that were depleted in the reduced-calorie state.

It also cranked up your hormone output (especially insulin and testosterone). It basically went from famine to feast, a VERY anabolic time in which you can get muscle growth almost without trying.

In THIS program, we take advantage of that effect (the "Slingshot Effect") to basically EXPLODE your muscle mass VERY quickly. We're going to put you in a low-calorie state for seven days, which is enough time for the body to adapt and set up the slingshot. Then we're going to turn you loose. It's like the diet phase pulls back on the slingshot, and the muscle-growth phase lets it go, rocketing your muscle growth forward.

This is a VERY powerful effect on its own, but we're going to add a few MORE wrinkles to really maximize the hormonal and metabolic effects you get from it.

And here's the other bonus: While you'll be doing a "diet" phase primarily to set up the muscle-building phases of the program, this diet has the added benefit of being a very effective way to control body fat gains while you are building muscle.

I'm sure you've experienced other muscle-building programs that simply rely on excess calories to support muscle growth. Nothing wrong with that except that you have a tendency to store any extra calories (above what's required for muscle growth) as fat. By starting out with a diet, you actually drop some fat at the start. When you start eating more in the following weeks, you're already ahead of the game.

But please note, I am NOT saying you won't gain any body fat when you're in your muscle-building phases. Honestly, it's quite likely that you WILL because I DO recommend that you eat an excess of calories to build maximum muscle. But the approaches you use in this program will serve to MINIMIZE fat gain.

Effective muscle building DOES require an excess of calories. To ensure you're getting enough calories, it's better to eat a little more than you need rather than less. You must give your body the nutrients and calories it needs to build the muscle.

How We Set Up the Slingshot Effect

We set up this effect not only with a caloric deficit (eating less), but also by limiting nutrients. The nutrients you eat have a HUGE effect on the body's hormone levels. By manipulating your nutrients during the first week, we're going to MAGNIFY the Slingshot Effect even MORE.

We'll be following what I call Macronutrient Rotation. In simple terms, during this first week, you'll rotate the three major macronutrients (protein, fat, and carbohydrates) in and out of your diet in very specific intervals by eating specific foods. It may sound complex, but the theory is simple. I'll present a basic run-through here, and there are web addresses to more specific information about each phase of the nutritional program below.

The bulk of the first week is low-carb eating. This stabilizes blood sugar levels and burns up your body's glycogen stores (usually a preferred fuel for muscles). Eating low-carb also increases insulin sensitivity (which we're going to take HUGE advantage of as we move into the next phase of the program). On these two days, the training we do will get rid of stored glycogen very quickly and give your metabolism a boost.

The third day of the program is a quick switch to low-fat, higher-carb eating. Because this is a muscle-building program, we don't want the body to get TOO depleted and start breaking down muscle tissue. The higher-carb day breaks things up and starts to refill glycogen levels. But the key HERE is that we're STILL keeping the calories down. This isn't a "real" carb-loading day; it's a quick punch to keep your metabolism moving. It's also a complete day of rest.

On the fourth and fifth days, it's back to strict, low-carb eating. On these two days, training is designed to elicit a large lactic-acid response, which will give you a surge of growth hormone. GH is more effective when insulin is not present, so what better time to promote it than when you are not eating carbs!

On the sixth day, we eat ONLY protein—no carbs or fats. Why? The body has been relying on fat for energy for most of the past week. By taking away dietary fat, only body fat is left. Also, eating only protein means a LARGE drop in caloric intake. We're setting your body up for a big rebound with this day.

On the seventh day, we switch again. This time, you'll be eating ONLY fruit. Nothing else. This is a zero-protein day to help set up the increased calorie and protein eating to come. It's also a great digestive system cleansing, which can really help with nutrient absorption when you start eating more again. I'll tell you more about the REAL muscle-building power of protein deprivation in the Nutrient Isolation section.

After that seventh day, we are ready to roll. The next day, you're going to immediately increase your caloric intake a LOT. You're also going to load up on protein (to take advantage of the previous day's protein deprivation). For the next few days, your body will be MADLY storing everything it can get its hands on.

So oblige it and feed the machine! You should see a substantial increase in bodyweight over the course of this week. The training during this week is the 5-Day Structural Attack, which is one of THE most effective muscle-building techniques I've found. Combine it with the big-time influx of nutrients and you are set up for a RAPID AND MASSIVE gain in muscle and strength.

IMPORTANT: Before I tell you exactly how to do these phases, please keep in mind that I am not a medical doctor or a nutritionist. This information is for educational purposes only, and you should always consult your physician before making any major changes to your diet.

Week 1

Low-Carb Eating

This week, you will first deprive your body of carbs (bread, potatoes, pasta, fruit, sugars, etc.), forcing it to rely more on fat for energy. This also sets up a desperate need for carbs.

Note: You will also learn how to adapt the low-carb regimen if you have difficulties with very low-carb eating.

Nutrient Isolation Days

In the two nutrient isolation days, you first deprive your body of both carbs and fats, forcing your body to burn body fat for energy. Next, you deprive it of both protein and fats, setting up a desperate need for protein.

Weeks 2-4

Eating for Mass

Here you not only provide that protein in mass quantities (it will be stored as muscle), you also provide plenty of carbohydrates and overall calories.

Supplements

In this section, you will learn which supplements are useful and EXACTLY how to take them to maximize your results and see dramatic changes in body composition.

Post-Workout Nutrition

Find out what you need to eat after a workout to take full advantage of both the training and nutritional guidelines you are following. Without proper post-workout nutrition, you could be throwing results away.

A Note About Alcohol Use

Alcohol use should be eliminated or greatly minimized while you are on the Muscle Explosion Program. Alcohol is known for its detrimental effects on both fat-burning and muscle-building hormones, and its use can severely hamper your results. If you are serious about getting the best results possible, save your alcohol use for when you're not on the program.

Week 1: Low-Carb Eating

Low-carb eating normally has no place in a muscle-building program. I'll tell you that right now. The reason is that it dramatically reduces the body's insulin secretion. Insulin is a key anabolic hormone. Without adequate insulin levels, your muscle cells simply don't absorb nutrients as efficiently. When used properly, though, low-carb eating is a great tool to maximize that Slingshot Effect.

If you've heard of the Atkins Diet, you're familiar with low-carb eating. The premise is simple: By depriving your body of its preferred fuel (carbohydrates), you force it to rely on fat stores for energy.

This approach works extremely well for short periods, which is exactly why you will follow it for just a few days. I will tell you how it works, how to do it, and the one reason you shouldn't do it for long.

How It Works

The benefits of the low-carb diet have very much to do with the stability of your blood sugar. When you don't add sugar or carbohydrates to your body, your blood sugar is very stable, limiting insulin production and allowing your fat stores to be mobilized easier. Reducing the carbs available to your body forces it to rely more on stored fats for energy. It's theorized that this new reliance on fat for energy increases the production of fat-burning enzymes in the body—a very good thing for dieters!

Another reason low-carb diets work is that eliminating a major nutrient from your diet automatically reduces the amount of calories you take in. Naturally, you can easily make this number up with fat calories; but studies have shown a tendency for people to naturally reduce caloric intake on a low-carb diet even when given free rein to eat as much as they want.

This can have a downside, however, as a person can minimize their appetite too much, artificially lowering their metabolism. You definitely want to avoid this.

It is important to note, too, that even if you are eating low-carb, you still need to keep an eye on total calories. If you are taking in more calories than your body burns, you won't lose fat regardless. This is the false assumption often associated with the low-carb diet. You really can't eat as much as you want. We always want to maintain some caloric deficit. The metabolic effects of this program mean you don't have to reduce your calories much, however.

As I've mentioned before, this reduced-calorie situation coupled with lowered insulin secretion is going to set up the body not only for the caloric overload of the following week, but also for the CARB overload of the following week. Because when you've deprived your body of carbs, it desperately wants to get carbs back into the system. When it does get carbs back in the system, it OVERLOADS the glycogen stores in the muscles with far more than it normally carries. This is called carb-loading.

This is a HIGHLY anabolic process that takes along water, protein, and other nutrients as well. Bottom line: You're going to gain a LOT very quickly.

How to Do It

To eat a low-carb diet, you must reduce your carbohydrate intake to 30 to 50 grams per day. You can certainly go below this as well.

I normally recommend shooting for 30 grams a day, as extra carbs have a way of sneaking into foods. Aiming for the low end means you'll be much more likely to stay within the proper range.

This is done by eliminating or drastically reducing intake of carbohydrate-containing foods such as breads, fruits, rice, pasta, cereals, grains, sugars, etc.

You will focus on eating low-carb foods such as meats, fish, poultry, healthy oils (fish oil, flax, hemp, olive, etc.), vegetables, salads, and cheese.

It is essential that you read labels and know exactly what you're eating when you go low-carb. There can be hidden carbs in foods you may think of as low-carb.

To further help you in this phase of the program, here are Web sites for more detailed information. These sites explain in great detail how to follow a low-carb diet. You'll find meal plans, charts of the number of carbs in certain foods, foods to avoid, etc.:

www.lowcarb.ca

www.lowcarbfriends.com

www.lowcarbluxury.com

www.atkins.com

My personal preference when eating low-carb is to focus primarily on natural, low-carb foods such as meats, eggs, cheese, vegetables, salads, and healthy oils, rather than foods that are manufactured to be low-carb.

To maximize the fat loss and health benefits, add in healthy oils such as fish oil, flax oil, olive oil, etc., for energy.

I prefer to save the majority of my carbs each day for a post-workout protein shake, as these carbs give you the most bang for your buck. I take about 20 grams of carbs right after a workout, with the other 10 grams spread throughout the day. On non-training days, spread the 30 grams out wherever you like.

I personally recommend AGAINST eating bacon, sausage, and other processed, fatty meats regularly, even on a low carb diet. They are OK as an occasional treat, but don't rely on them as a regular part of your diet. Being on a low-carb diet should not be a license to eat garbage food. What you eat still needs to be processed by your body, after all, and junk is still junk!

Also, it is important to minimize fat intake following your workouts, even while on a higher-fat diet like this. Post-workout fat intake has been shown to decrease circulating growth hormone levels by HALF [Reference 10]. Eat low-fat, low-carb foods following your workout to maximize the effects of your training.

In Week 1 you will eat low-carb for four out of five days. This sets you up for the All-Protein Day and the Zero-Protein Day, which will both be explained in detail in the Nutrient Isolation Days section.

Net Carbs, Effective Carbs, and Impact Carbs—Good or Bad?

While keeping track of net carbs, effective carbs, and impact carbs may be good for some, I personally DO NOT recommend frequently eating foods that rely on these definitions and alterations. Naturally low-carb foods, in my opinion, are simply better for you.

The less processing a food has been through, the easier it is for your body to work with. Manufactured low-carb foods are, in many cases, just the same junk food repackaged in a low-carb format to give the appearance of being healthy. My recommendation is to eliminate or minimize these foods. The body simply wasn't designed to digest the large amounts of sugar alcohol that most of these rely on.

Why You Shouldn't Do Low-Carb for Long

The low-carb approach is not the easiest to follow for long periods of time, nor is it the most effective. Most people are simply not used to eating foods such as meats, eggs, fish, and salad with nothing on the side. It can be hard to stick to this diet in the long term. That's not really an issue with the Muscle Explosion Program, as you'll only be doing it for a few days. But I want to be sure you get this info about low-carb eating in general.

As far as results go, you will get fast results at first. You will lose several pounds of water right away as the carbs are burned and the water associated with them gets flushed out. After that, you will get into more fat burning.

If you keep up with this eating style, however, your body eventually starts to slow your metabolism. Your appetite will decrease. Results will slow and maybe even stop! When you're not getting any results, it's tough to deprive yourself of carb-containing foods.

But with this program, when we switch up the eating the following week, your metabolism will roar back into overdrive.

Carb Tapering: An Alternative to Low-Carb Eating

Not everyone has an easy time with a low-carb diet. In fact, some people can't do it for medical reasons. Therefore, I want to provide you with an adaptation called Carb-Tapering.

Here's how it works: Instead of completely cutting carbs from your diet, you will taper them down over the course of the day. You will eat most of your carbs early in the day, gradually reducing them as the day goes on. Your last meal of the day should contain very few if any carbs, and definitely don't eat any carbs in the evening.

Eat lower-fat foods when you eat your earlier meals. Your later, lower-carb meals can contain larger amounts of fats, preferably healthy fats such as fish oil, olive oil, flax oil, etc.

If this approach is better for you, follow it in place of the regular low-carb diet during Week 1, including the only protein day, as explained above. Remember, though, that while this eating style will work reasonably well, it is a compromise and won't get results as good as if you were following the regular low-carb plan.

Be ABSOLUTELY SURE you are eating fewer overall calories. That is critical to making the Slingshot Effect work most effectively.

Weeks 2 Through 4: Eating for Mass

We've finished with the strict portions of the diet phase. Now we get to the fun part, where you get to really EAT.

But, ironically enough, some people actually DREAD this part. Why? Because the amount of food most programs require you to eat can be HARD to fit in your belly, especially if you don't have a big appetite to begin with. It's a problem that's more common than you might think, and I'm going to tell you my solution for it. Because, to really gain substantial muscle mass, you DO need to take in a lot of calories and nutrients.

Let's continue where we left off. You've just finished the all-fruit day, and you're starting your first day of high-calorie eating.

You definitely want to eat a substantial amount of food, especially on training days. We're looking to load up on nutrients, so your caloric intake should be at least 300 to 500 calories (preferably more) above your "maintenance" value (the amount you eat when you're not really training specifically for muscle growth or eating for fat loss, but just trying to keep things as they are).

Protein, Carbs, and Fats: How Much of Each to Eat

During the three-week, muscle-building phase of the program, DO NOT be afraid of eating fat. It is more calorie-dense than any other nutrient. I'm not saying go out of your way to get it, but don't be afraid to eat a juicy steak and put some butter on your mashed potatoes. During these three weeks, the training is tough and your body needs those calories to recover and grow.

If you try to eat too "clean" (in this case, low-fat), you will compromise your results by not giving your body adequate calories. Also, you will shoot yourself in the foot hormonally. Testosterone levels decrease when you eat a low-fat diet. Sad, but true. By keeping your fat intake moderate instead of low, you will support testosterone production. This is absolutely CRITICAL to gaining muscle mass and strength. The higher your testosterone levels, the better your recovery will be.

When it comes to carbs, you want to really load up, especially on the first few days of this phase of the program. Your body is madly scooping up and storing all the carbs it can. The more you provide, the more it will store.

As for protein, as I mentioned previously, you want to really load up. Take in at least one gram of protein per pound of bodyweight on each of the first few days of the program (more is better). This means a 200-pound person should eat 200 grams of protein per day. You can taper that down after a few days, but I like to recommend keeping the one gram per pound rule through this phase. Your body needs a LOT of protein to recover from the training you're going to put it through.

The ratio of calories per food group will vary. In fact, I prefer not to nail down a specific ratio but rather focus first on getting plenty of protein, next on getting plenty of carbs, and finally on not restricting fat intake. The ratios then take care of themselves.

But if you are a numbers person, here you go: 25 percent to 35 percent of calories from protein, another 25 percent to 35 percent from fat, and 45 percent to 55 percent from carbs. These ranges are VERY inexact, so don't base your life on them.

How to Eat for Mass without Constantly Stuffing Yourself Silly

I'm not a big fan of stuffing yourself full of food every meal of the day to gain mass. That not only keeps you feeling continuously stuffed, it is more likely to make you gain fat as you go through the program.

To get the best results possible while keeping fat gain to a minimum, I recommend timing your food intake to coincide with time of day and your training. It's a simple concept, and one that I've found to be VERY effective for really piling on muscle mass while keeping fat gain low.

Your biggest meal of the day should be the one following your training session for the day. THAT is when your body is really primed to use the nutrients you put in. I've found that you can eat upwards of one-third to one-half of your day's total calorie intake in your post-workout meal and not gain significant fat. Overfeeding this way is also VERY anabolic. The massive influx of nutrients gives your body a signal that it can start packing on the muscle mass without worrying about preparing for a famine.

Your NEXT biggest meal should be breakfast. You've just had a long overnight fast and your body is ready to get some nutrition in. It will process and use everything efficiently.

Your remaining meals should be small to moderate in size—no stuffing yourself. The smaller meals will help your body process the nutrients more efficiently, which means you don't have to eat as much. Note, however, that these small meals should involve high-quality food. I don't mean a bag of chips. A small meal might be a piece of fish and potatoes with veggies.

The bottom line is this: Don't stuff yourself the whole day through. Eat a larger meal when you have a REASON, like waking up in the morning or after a hard workout. You'll get the benefits of high-calorie eating without the increase in fat that you normally see.

What to Eat for Mass:

Get a pen and a piece of paper and draw four vertical lines down the page.

In the first column, write down all the protein foods you like to eat. (for example, beef, chicken, eggs, fish, etc.). In the second column, write down all the carb-containing foods you like to eat (potatoes, rice, bread, pasta, etc.). In the third column, write down all the fruits, vegetables, and salad stuff you like (apples, bananas, broccoli, carrots, greens, berries, etc.).

In the fourth column, write down all the foods that are a mix of the others or are processed (for example, lasagna, hamburgers, casseroles, etc.).

In the fifth column, list all the foods that don't really fit into the other categories because they're basically junk food (pizza, desserts, etc.).

Now here are the rules:

1. At least 75 percent of your food intake should come from the first three columns. A rule of thumb I like to use is one protein source, one carb source and one fruit/veggie/salad source in each meal.

2. Next, no more than 20 percent of your food intake should come from the mixed/processed column.

3. Finally, not more than 5 percent of your food intake should come from the junk food column. You can consider these as "cheat" meals if you like, or just consider them as part of the eating program. Sometimes, when I'm eating for mass, I just feel like I need a big "calorie bomb" pizza to really get things fueled up.

These rules mean the majority of your food is coming from unprocessed, natural foods, but you don't have to be a saint about what you're eating.

Food from the last two columns, while not ideal, CAN provide a lot of calories and definitely increase your eating enjoyment, which is important, too. You can also add foods in the appropriate columns as you find new things you like.

Now that you know WHAT to eat, it's just a matter of eating at the appropriate times and in appropriate quantities! THAT is your meal plan.

My Tips on Eating for Mass

Here are some more tips and reminders as you go through Weeks 2 through 4:

- Eat a generous amount of protein daily to take advantage of the protein-deprivation day (approximately one gram of protein per pound of bodyweight per day). You can also calculate this formula based on lean bodyweight, the theory being that fat is not metabolically active and doesn't require protein to maintain itself. While this is true, calculating based on your total bodyweight will make sure that you eat MORE protein, which is what we're looking to do in this phase. That's why I prefer to compute it this way.

- Try to primarily eat foods that are less processed. They are healthier, and easier for your body to digest and work with.

- I find it's also best to keep the number of ingredients you eat in any given meal to a minimum. The fewer the number of different foods your body has to work on processing, the more efficient it will be. What do you think is easier to process, a bowl of oatmeal or toast, juice, eggs, milk, cereal, and fruit? The rule of thumb I like to follow is one protein source, one complex carb source, and one vegetable source (though you CAN eat more than one vegetable source without a problem).

- Try to eat fairly frequently throughout the day. This stimulates your metabolism to a greater degree than fewer but larger meals. Every time you eat, your metabolism is stimulated. That being said, it's perfectly fine if you can only get in three meals a day. Sometimes, that's all I can do. I wake up, have a protein shake, eat a BIG breakfast, have lunch in the early afternoon, train late in the afternoon, then have a BIG post-workout meal. For me, this system works like a charm. I get great results and I don't get hungry. If you can eat five or six meals a day, go for it. If you can't, don't worry about it.

- Drink plenty of water! This is extremely important in all phases but especially when your target is adding muscle. Water is what your muscles are primarily made of. Your muscles also need to be well hydrated to function properly AND to grow. Muscle growth occurs in the soup inside your muscles. Without enough water, the soup gets thick, and muscle growth and repair slow down! You should drink water VERY frequently throughout the day.

- Don't be afraid of leftovers. When eating for mass, make a LOT when you make something. That way, you'll always have leftovers that you can eat the next day without having to cook again.

Post-Workout Nutrition

What is your post-workout nutritional regimen?

If you answered "nothing," you are cheating yourself out of results that are rightfully yours. You may be wasting as much as 50 percent of your effort in the gym by not maximizing your post-workout nutrition.

When you train, your body burns fats and carbohydrates for energy and breaks down your muscle tissue. Immediately after a workout, the body has an enhanced ability to utilize nutrients such as glucose and protein to rebuild and recover from your exercise.

This essentially means your body is turbocharged and ready to grow. This period of power lasts for approximately four hours after a workout, hence the common name for it: the Four-Hour Window of Opportunity.

Taking in nutrients immediately after exercise helps you recover faster and feel better after a workout. It can help you not only gain muscle faster, but also keep your metabolism fueled so that you lose fat at a faster rate, too.

What happens if you don't eat immediately following a training session? Let me put it this way: It's definitely a situation you want to avoid.

First, your body starts breaking down muscle tissue in undamaged areas in order to get raw materials to help repair the areas you've just worked. Over time, this will result in a loss of muscle from your whole body.

Stress hormones in the body (primarily a hormone called cortisol) speed this process along. The stress hormones are produced because working out is a stress on the body. It's a totally natural, but results-stopping reaction. How do you control the effects of cortisol? You eat as soon as you can.

And please don't think that waiting an hour after your workout will result in burning off more fat when you finally do eat. It really causes you to burn off muscle tissue. Your body will do whatever it has to do to rebuild itself, including breaking down protein from other areas to repair the just-used parts.

What do you eat after a workout to maximize your results? Both protein and carbohydrates are CRITICAL for fast recovery.

Protein

Immediately following a workout (within a few minutes of its completion), take in some protein. This gives your body something to rebuild with. The easiest, best way to do this is in the form of a protein powder (whey is an excellent choice).

Drinking milk post-workout is OK, but not the best choice. You want to get protein into your body as quickly as possible. Milk has to first curdle in the stomach, THEN get digested slowly, bit by bit, before amino acids can be used. You won't get protein quickly enough.

I prefer not to take in protein right before a workout. Why? If it doesn't get completely digested, it will sit in your gut and possibly cause bloating.

Try to get at least 30 to 40 grams of protein in as soon as you can after you're finished training. Other examples of protein foods include eggs, poultry, fish, lean meat, or soy products.

Carbohydrates

If you are in the muscle-building weeks of the program, take in 60 to 100 grams of carbohydrates to help the body refuel. Your body is most efficient at rebuilding its carbohydrate stores immediately after a workout. It's important to take advantage of this. If you are in the low-carb phase of the program, limit your carb intake to 20 grams. Immediately after your workout is the most effective time to take your carbs for the day when eating low-carb.

Right after a workout is one of the few times when simple carbs (sugary, quick-to-digest carbs) are actually very useful. The simple carbs will help your body make use of the other nutrients you are putting in by raising insulin levels. The insulin helps shuttle these nutrients into the cells. Your body is more sensitive to carbs when you're on a low-carb diet, so you don't need nearly as many to get a reaction.

Healthy carbs to eat post-workout include juices, fruits, and sports drinks. Flavored yogurt is another excellent post-workout food snack. It contains carbs, protein, and calcium all in one.

Fats

It is important to minimize your fat intake following your workouts. Post-workout fat intake has been shown to decrease circulating growth hormone levels by HALF [Reference 10]. This is not something we want to happen. That being said, a small dose of a healthy fat, such as flax oil, can have positive effects on recovery.

Post-Workout Meal

About one hour or so after your workout is when to have your BIG post-workout meal.

Take in a high-quality protein and a good supply of carbohydrates such as grains, potatoes, or cereals. At this time, the body has settled down from the stress of the workout and is looking to rebuild. It's fine to take in fats now, too. If you're looking to get as much from your workouts as you possibly can, post-workout nutrition is critical.

Supplementation

Supplements can really help maximize your results on the Muscle Explosion Program. I'm recommending basic supplements—the ones that have been PROVEN to work. You don't need anything fancy to really get results (contrary to what you might read in magazines that rely on supplement advertising to stay in business). The "latest" things usually create a great big hole in the wallet, and that's money better spent on getting yourself better quality food!

How you use these supplements and when is what really gets you the results! I'll go through what to use, when to use it, and why. The big thing to keep in mind here is that supplements are the icing on the cake. They're NOT the driving force behind your results. Training and nutrition are the REAL driving forces behind results. Supplements help, but they won't make up for useless training or terrible nutrition.

I'm not against TRYING new supplements. Not at all. If you want to try some of the new things coming out, definitely go for it. Do your research first, though. What I recommend is trying ONE new supplement at a time so you know if and what worked. If you try five new things at once, who knows what did what! The cheapest thing you bought may be the one that got you the result.

Take ALL advertising with a grain of salt. That huge guy you see in the picture? Chances are he didn't get that way simply because he took a couple of creatine pills every day. It's good to get excited about trying new things. I try new supplements all the time. Keep an open mind, but keep your eyes open, too.

Let's get started!

Multivitamins

A good multivitamin is a critical part of ANYBODY'S supplement routine. I don't care how well you eat, you simply CAN'T get optimal levels of nutrients through food alone. I'm not talking RDI (Recommended Daily Intake) or anything like that. The RDI is the level necessary to prevent deficiency. I don't know about you, but I'd rather take enough of something to actually HAVE an effect, not prevent a deficiency.

Plus, most food simply does not have enough nutrients in it these days to allow even the healthiest eater to get optimal amounts of vitamins and minerals, even when eating regular meals. Think of a multivitamin as an insurance policy. It helps protect you from any deficiencies you might not know about.

And if someone tells you all you'll get is expensive urine, tell them your urine is worth it. You'd rather have "expensive" urine now than INCREDIBLY expensive urine later in life when the doctors tell you that you need a $90-a-pill bone-loss treatment because you didn't take in enough calcium earlier in life.

Multivitamins are especially important during dieting because of reduced nutrient intake, especially during the low-carb phase of this diet. But you ALSO need them when training to gain muscle. There are LOTS of chemical processes in the body that require ample quantities of vitamins and minerals. If you don't have them available, your body will simply shut the growth process down.

Going back to our earlier house analogy, what happens if you are putting up the frame and you run out of nails? Substituting tiny nails won't work. They'll put a complete STOP to the building process, just as missing tiny amounts of some vitamins and minerals will stop your muscle growth.

Don't take generic, low-quality multivitamins either. You may as well be swallowing little rocks for all the nutrients you will get out of them.

Most vitamins (including popular brand names) that come in tablet form are so compressed that they can't be broken down even by stomach acid.

Look for multivitamins in capsule or gelcap form. These are the most absorbable.

The multivitamin I'm currently taking is "Eco Green Multi" from NOW Foods. You can order it online at *www.fitstep.com/goto/multivitamin.htm.*

Protein

Protein is the basic building block of muscle tissue. Without enough protein, all your training efforts are for naught because your body won't have the raw materials to recover and rebuild.

Protein is readily available in food, but protein-containing foods are not always the most convenient to prepare or eat. When was the last time you packed some scrambled eggs into your backpack for a snack? Plus, post-workout, you want to get protein into the muscles as quickly as possible. The body digests something like whey protein MUCH faster.

When to Take Protein in the Phases

Protein can and should be taken during all phases of the program except the Zero-Protein Day. (Guess that makes sense!)

To take full advantage of the effect of the protein starvation day, try Protein Loading on the first day of the muscle-building phase (Week 2).

Protein Loading is simple: Take one scoop of protein powder every two hours on the hour while you are awake (aside from mealtimes and training times). If your protein powder gives you 20 grams per scoop, this could mean as much as 160 grams of extra protein or more! Remember, at this point your body is sucking up and storing every available gram of protein you give it. This helps maximize the effectiveness.

Protein Loading need only be done on the first day of Week 2, but keep up a regular, fairly high protein intake otherwise. Here's the when, why, and how of effective daily protein supplementation, ranked in order of importance.

1. Immediately After a Workout

If you take protein only once per day, this is the absolute best time to take it. Immediately after you finish your workout, your body needs raw materials to rebuild and recover with. If you don't supply them through eating, your body will break down muscle from elsewhere to rebuild the damaged areas. This is counterproductive.

By taking in some protein (30 to 50 grams or so) within minutes after exercise, you provide the raw materials your body needs.

2. First Thing in the Morning

Immediately upon waking, or as soon after that as you can, take a scoop of protein powder. Your body has just been through a fast of eight hours or more, and it's hungry for nutrients. Feed your body!

Protein powder is more quickly assimilated than solid food and gets into your muscles faster. This protein shot gives your metabolism a boost, and that can help with fat loss. Be sure to follow it with a good breakfast, of course.

3. An Hour After a Workout

About an hour after a workout, your body has settled down from the excitement and is ready to really start rebuilding. The protein that you took in immediately following the workout has been metabolized, and your body is looking for more. Another protein shake at this time is a good way to help speed recovery. You want to take in another 20 to 30 grams of protein now. This is also when you should be getting ready to have your post-workout meal.

4. Last Thing at Night

Prepare your body for the long overnight fast by giving it a little something to work with. A good combination before bed is to mix a scoop of whey protein with a small glass of milk.

Whey is what's known as a "fast" protein, meaning that it's digested quickly, while milk protein (casein) is a "slow" protein. At night, you want your protein to be metabolized slowly so your body gets a more even supply throughout the night. By mixing "fast" and "slow" proteins, you get the benefits of the higher-quality whey with the slower digestion time of the milk.

If you can get it, a straight milk protein or a protein blend supplement is even better. That way, you don't get the lactose that you do by adding in milk.

5. Between Meals

A quick protein shake can be a great snack between meals. It helps keep your body supplied with protein all day long.

This is especially useful if you go long periods between meals. It could mean the difference between losing muscle and building or keeping muscle!

6. With Meals
Taking a protein supplement with meals is a handy way to increase the protein content of the meal. This is a perfect balance to a meal that is somewhat lower in protein.

7. In the Middle of the Night
This is a trick bodybuilders sometimes use. It keeps your muscles supplied throughout the night. Keep a premixed protein shake beside your bed. Although some trainers set alarms to wake up to drink it, I prefer to have it there waiting just in case I wake up. I don't wake up on purpose. If I don't wake up, it's right there ready for me to drink first thing in the morning! This strategy is more targeted for muscle growth than fat loss.

NOTE: Taking Protein Before a Workout

Personally, I'm not a big fan of taking a protein shake before training. Some people do this thinking it will give them an energy boost or a head start for post-workout recovery. Instead, that shake often sits in the stomach and bloats them up. Valuable blood that should be going to working muscles gets sent to the digestive system to try to digest the shake.

That being said, if you DO want to take protein, take it 30 minutes or more before training so it can digest. Give it a try with a small protein shake to make sure you don't get any adverse effects.

And keep in mind, the growth hormone response to training is greater when you don't have food in your stomach. So DON'T take protein before training when on the low-carb phase of the diet. It will throw off the hormonal response and compromise results. For more information, go to *www.fitstep.com/goto/protein-finder.htm*.

Joint Supplements

Next on my list is a good joint supplement. Here's the deal: You can't train nearly as heavy when your joints are sore. And when you train heavy and don't take joint supplements, your joints WILL get sore.

I consider joint supplements ESSENTIAL for any serious trainer, more essential than creatine. Your joints have to last you a lifetime. Take care of them and they'll take care of you!

So, you MUST take a good joint supplement. Got that? You simply cannot get enough joint-support nutrients through diet alone. And, if you don't, your joints will eventually get ground down.

This is especially true when doing Partial and other training that directly targets the connective tissue. When you break down muscle tissue, you provide protein to help it rebuild. The same goes for joints and connective tissue. If you target them, you MUST support them nutritionally.

Here's my list of the top joint-support nutrients:

> *Glucosamine: 1,500 mg per day*
> *(500 mg taken three times a day is good.)*
> *Chondroitin: 400 to 600 mg per day*
> *MSM: 1 to 2 grams per day*
> *Hyaluronic Acid: follow label instructions*
> *Vitamin C: 1,000 to 5,000 mg per day*
> *Gelatin: 1 to 5 grams per day (varies)*
> *Calcium: 1,000 to 1,500 mg per day*

Check out *www.fitstep.com/goto/joints.htm.*

The product I use is Joint Care from Beverly International. It's a gelcap that has a good spectrum of the major joint-support nutrients.

Creatine: Monohydrate or Ethyl Ester

Creatine monohydrate is an excellent muscle-building supplement. It is completely safe for both men and women. Many scientific studies document its safety and effectiveness. It is a natural substance found primarily in red meat.

Using creatine can cause a rapid weight gain of three to 10 pounds during the loading phase, depending on the amount of muscle and water you are carrying. The bigger you are, the more weight you will gain. This weight is primarily in the form of more water in your muscles.

Creatine builds strength by increasing the amount of fuel available for muscle contractions. By increasing your available fuel, your body is able to lift more weight and do more reps. This, in turn, allows you to build muscle. Also, it's been theorized that the increased water levels in your muscles give them better leverage when performing exercises, leading to increased strength.

When to Take Creatine in the Phases

Creatine users typically load up for five days, then drop down to a maintenance dose to keep high levels in the muscles. If you are using Creatine Monohydrate, this is exactly what you'll do. If you are taking Creatine Ethyl Ester (a more absorbable form), there's no need to load up. Still, on the first day, I like to take multiple doses just to get more creatine into my body. It can give you a good kick-start.

On the first day of Week 2, you will start loading up on creatine. Take four doses of five grams (which is about a teaspoon) on all five days of the 5-Day Structural Attack. After that, drop down to a maintenance dose of one teaspoon per day.

Your doses can be taken any time during the day. I like to take mine according to my workout schedule. Take one dose about 45 minutes before training and one dose immediately AFTER, along with your post-workout shake. For the other two doses, I take one first thing in the morning and the other at any other convenient time between meals.

Week 2 of the program is the PERFECT time to start a loading phase. Your body is coming off the low-carb phase and will be more sensitive to the effects of insulin. By taking your creatine with a high-glycemic carbohydrate (which is what I recommend—I use a scoop of Tang drink mix myself. No need to get fancy), your body will not only release more insulin, it will be more sensitive to its effects, shuttling more creatine into your muscles.

You will be rapidly gaining muscle from the Protein Loading you'll be doing. Adding creatine to this mix will help that process move even FASTER.

Drink a LOT of water when loading up on creatine. Muscle cramping can occur if you don't. Plus, we WANT ample water available to maximize weight/water gain during this loading phase! During these few days, you should be practically SLOSHING.

During the rest of the program, the maintenance dose can be taken immediately after training. On "off" days, take it any time between meals or first thing in the morning.

Creatine Monohydrate vs. Creatine Ethyl Ester

These are the two major versions of creatine on the market today. Creatine monohydrate is the "old standard." It works like a charm for most people. But for some, it's not particularly absorbable and they may get gastrointestinal upset. These folks are known as "creatine non-responders." Monohydrate is the cheaper version of creatine and the most extensively studied. If you've used and gotten good results with it, continue to use it.

Creatine Ethyl Ester is a newer version. It is purported to be more absorbable. Therefore, you don't have to take it in such large doses. It tends to work for people who are typically monohydrate non-responders.

The creatine ethyl ester I've used is in a product called Hyper Gain. I find it VERY effective. To learn more about it and get a sample, go to www.fitstep.com/goto/hyper-gain.htm. For regular creatine,
visit www.fitstep.com/goto/creatine.htm.

Glutamine

Glutamine is a nonessential amino acid in the body, but it is also the most abundant amino acid in the body. Around 50 percent of the body's free amino acid pool consists of glutamine. I'm a big fan of glutamine use, especially when you are training hard and looking to make gains. I've been taking it regularly for years and find that when I don't, it really affects my recovery between workouts.

Taking extra glutamine has a variety of beneficial effects.

A dose of just two grams on an empty stomach has been shown to increase the level of circulating growth hormone. This is good because growth hormone promotes muscle growth and fat loss.

Supplementing with glutamine also means the body doesn't have to break down other amino acids to make it. Glutamine is a much-used amino acid, and if glutamine levels are low, the body will break down muscle protein to synthesize it. If you provide it, your body doesn't have to.

Glutamine supplements help support muscle growth if taken in doses of five grams or more at a time. This large amount is necessary to get enough past the digestive system to be of value. The gut sucks up glutamine like a sponge.

Other positive effects of glutamine include immune-system boosting, improved recovery, cell volumization, and enhancement of glycogen replenishment.

Glutamine attracts water much as creatine does. Thus, it has a cell-volumizing effect that is very anabolic. Remember, the more water you can get into your muscles cells, the better they'll grow.

The best times to take glutamine are first thing in the morning, right after a workout, and right before sleep.

Dosages can vary from two grams (minimum) to 10 to 15 grams or more. The larger doses should be used immediately after a workout to promote anabolism and minimize catabolism (muscle breakdown).

Personally, I take about 20 to 30 grams immediately after every workout. The more you can take in, the better (though I don't go above 40 grams per dose).

When to Take Glutamine in the Phases

Glutamine should be taken after every training session. It helps your body recover more quickly from the intense training you are doing. It will also help keep your immune system functioning at peak levels as you push yourself over the course of the program, especially toward the last few days of the 5-Day Structural Attack. This is a critical time. If your immune system is down, you're more likely to get sick. Glutamine is fuel for your immune system. I recommend taking it in greater quantities even when you're not on the program if you start feeling any sort of illness coming on.

In addition to taking it after every workout, you can also try Glutamine Loading on the first two days of Week 2, when you start taking creatine as well. Load up by taking four doses each day. Take five grams first thing in the morning and five grams an hour before training. Take 10 to 20 grams right after training and five grams right before bed. After these first two days, you can go back to taking it only after workouts.

Glutamine is easiest to take in powder form. Capsules are available, but you need to take so many to get results that it's just not worth it. Imagine glutamine coming in one gram or 500 mg pills and trying to take in 20 grams. That's 20 to 40 pills! Glutamine powder is your best bet. For info, check out *www.fitstep.com/goto/glutamine.htm*.
Personally, I use the AST Sports Science brand GL-3 in the 1,000 gram size. It's a good price for a quality product. Even when you take a boatload of it, it lasts a good long time and is well worth it.

Minerals, Vitamins and Miscellaneous

I'll tell you right now, there is nothing glamorous about taking minerals and vitamins. You will NEVER see a full-page ad in Muscle & Fitness for the latest calcium supplement or see Mr. Olympia plugging a vitamin B complex.

But simple, basic nutrients like minerals and vitamins are absolutely CRITICAL for EVERYBODY who trains with weights. I'm going to mention a few of the major ones you need to take in sufficient amounts to make a BIG, FAST difference in your training.

You can get pretty much any of these things at any health food store or GNC (General Nutrition Center) but I prefer to buy online. It keeps prices quite a bit lower.

Calcium

Calcium makes up the majority of your body's mineral weight (your bones). It's VERY important to take supplemental calcium. Your body simply doesn't absorb it well from most foods. You may drink lots of milk, but not much of that calcium is actually getting absorbed.

Ideally, you should take 1,000 to 1,500 mg per day. This will support bone health and a host of other processes that require calcium (including blood clotting, nerve function, and muscle contraction). If you don't get enough calcium, you compromise your long-term health. If you don't provide enough in your diet, your body will PULL IT OUT OF YOUR BONES to get it.

Calcium excretion actually INCREASES when you're eating a high-protein diet, making it doubly important for those looking to increase muscle mass to get plenty of calcium.

Vitamin D is required for optimal calcium absorption, so look for it in any calcium supplements you purchase. Be sure that you don't take more than 2,000 mg of calcium per day. Also, calcium intake should be balanced with magnesium intake (more on this below). The ratio should be 2:1 calcium to magnesium, meaning you should take 1,000 mg of calcium for every 500 mg of magnesium.

The best sources of supplemental calcium (in terms of absorbability) are calcium citrate and calcium citrate malate. Coral calcium also is said to be highly absorbable.

Many calcium products also include magnesium in them.
www.fitstep.com/goto/calcium.htm

Magnesium

Magnesium is one of THE most important minerals in the body. It is essential for more than 300 body processes! Yet it is often missing from both food and supplement regimens. While true magnesium deficiency is rare, you can benefit greatly from ingesting optimal levels. Magnesium is critical for cellular energy production, as well as body structure (bones especially) and the healing process.

Bottom line, if you're not getting enough magnesium, your strength will suffer. When you start getting optimal levels, you will probably notice a strength increase fairly rapidly.

Magnesium intake should ideally be balanced with calcium intake (the 2:1 ratio mentioned above). Minimum intake for a healthy adult is 300 to 400 mg per day (depending on bodyweight). You can take an additional 300 to 400 mg per day supplemental. What's the easiest way to tell if you're taking too much? Larger doses of magnesium have a laxative effect.

The easiest way to purchase and take magnesium is in a formula combined with calcium. That way, you just take one pill instead of doubling up. The citrate form of magnesium is one of the better absorbed.
www.fitstep.com/goto/calcium.htm

Zinc

Zinc is another critical mineral. It acts as a catalyst for many of the body's chemical reactions and processes.It also plays a critical role in the structure of proteins and cell membranes, and it's important for immune system function and anabolic hormone production (for example, testosterone).

Most multivitamins have some zinc, but you may benefit from taking a 25 to 50 mg zinc supplement on its own. DO NOT go above 150 mg per day for more than a few days. Zinc is one of the few minerals that can produce adverse reactions in relatively low overdoses. More is not better in this case.
www.fitstep.com/goto/zinc.htm

Vitamin C

Vitamin C is a totally unglamorous supplement that can have tremendous effects on your training and health. It is a MUST-HAVE, in my opinion. The amount necessary to stave off deficiency is about 60 mg per day. The amount for optimal health and performance is MUCH greater, especially when you are training your muscles hard and working on connective tissue.

Vitamin C is an essential component in the synthesis of collagen, which basically is what connective tissue is made of.

Without enough Vitamin C, collagen formation will grind down. For our purposes, we want to ensure we're getting PLENTY. Personally, I take about 3,000 to 5,000 mg per day. The good thing about Vitamin C is that it's water-soluble. Excess levels are easily and quickly flushed from the body.

Another important function of Vitamin C is as an antioxidant. It's very effective at quashing free radicals, which are a BIG concern when training hard. To prevent cell damage, antioxidant intake is vital.

And we can't forgot the effects of Vitamin C supplementation on cortisol levels. Cortisol is the stress hormone associated with stress and muscle breakdown. Three 1,000 mg doses of Vitamin C a day can decrease cortisol levels very effectively, which helps with staying anabolic. Think you're a hard gainer? Maybe you're not getting enough Vitamin C.

Lastly, Vitamin C taken before a workout (500 to 1,000 mg) can help reduce muscle soreness, which is VERY useful on this program, especially during the 5-Day Structural Attack.

You can take pretty much any version of Vitamin C. There's no research proving any one form is better than any other. *www.fitstep.com/goto/vitaminc.htm*

Fish Oil/Krill Oil

Fish oil and krill oil, which is thought by some to be better than fish oil, are an excellent supplement for bodybuilding and overall health. The active ingredients you get are EPA and DHA.

They benefit many areas of the body, including cell membrane structure and function, the nervous system, vision, and the heart and circulatory system. EPA and DHA act as anti-inflammatory agents, making them beneficial when training hard.

Taking three to five grams of fish oil a day is fine. You can generally get it in one gram capsules, which are preferred over taking the liquid. I recommend Nordic Naturals. *www.fitstep.com/goto/fish-oil.htm*

How to Take All These Supplements

Having all these supplements is one thing. Taking them all properly is another! Here's a quick guide to help you get it right.

1. **Multivitamin**
   Ideally, take this in divided doses two or three times a day, for example, morning, post-workout, and last thing at night.

2. **Protein**
   Post-workout, first thing in the morning, with meals, between meals.

3. **Joint Supplements**
   Take two or three times a day, for example, morning, post-workout, last thing at night.

4. Creatine

Load up at the start of Week 2. Then keep up with a maintenance dose for the remainder of the program. No creatine during Week 1.

5. Glutamine

Take 10 to 20 grams after every workout. You can load up on the first two days of Week 2. No glutamine on the Zero-Protein Day.

6. Calcium/Magnesium

Take two or three times a day in divided doses, for example, morning, post-workout, and night.

7. Zinc

Just once later in evening. (Take it with other vitamins last thing at night.)

8. Vitamin C

Take three times a day in divided doses (1,000 mg each time). Also 500 to 1,000 mg 45 minutes before training.

9. Fish Oil

Take two or three times a day in divided doses (one to three grams each dose).

You don't NEED to take ALL of these supplements to get results with the program. But, at the very least, I suggest a good multivitamin and a joint-support supplement. These are basic. Next in order of importance are protein, glutamine, creatine, calcium/magnesium, Vitamin C, fish oil, and zinc.

Once you have your basics taken care of, if you wish, you can try some "exotic" supplements to see how they work for you.

Bottom line, you'll get better results from your training and nutrition if you focus your supplementation on SUPPORTING the process rather than having supplements try to BE the driving force behind your results. Supplements won't lift that heavy barbell for you. And lifting that heavy barbell is what REALLY drives your results forward.

Caloric Intake

I'm going to start this section by letting you in on one of my dirty little secrets: I've NEVER counted calories in my life. I only measure food to figure out how much water to put in my oatmeal in the morning or to count the number of potatoes I have on my plate. I don't weigh food to determine how many calories it contains.

I HAVE added up my daily caloric intake ONCE, though, just out of curiosity. I did it during a MASSIVE eating cycle. Turns out the number was 8,500 calories in one day!

But now I'm going to tell you WHY I've never counted calories in my life.

I have a hard enough time finding time to cook and prepare food, never mind trying to figure out exactly how much of it I should be eating.

I learned long ago that if I want to lose fat, I have to eat LESS. And if I want to gain muscle, I have to eat MORE.

WHAT you eat and WHEN you eat are just as important as HOW MUCH you eat.

I like to keep things simple when it comes to nutrition. So, when it comes time to figure out exactly how much food you need to eat during this program, trust your instincts. I use my body and my results as a guide rather than counting calories.

When you're doing the low-carb, low-calorie diet phase, don't eat very much. It's that simple. Naturally, don't starve yourself. Be sure you're eating a decent amount of food and getting good nutrition, but just don't eat a lot. You're only going to be doing this low-calorie eating for a week, and the MAIN IDEA is to deprive and deplete yourself. No real tricks here: just don't eat very much.

If you get hungry during this phase, don't freak out and think you're suddenly going to lose all your muscle mass. That won't happen. Drink a glass of water, eat a few almonds, and let yourself be hungry for a little while. It's not going to kill you. This week, let that hunger build. You're telling your body there's a famine. Then, when you feast, it will respond BIG TIME.

When you switch over to the high-calorie phase, you eat a lot. Simple again! Dramatically increasing your caloric and nutrient intake is going to set off that cascade of anabolic hormones that will shoot your muscle growth through the roof!

In this phase, if you find your bodyweight isn't increasing as you go, just eat even more.

The Harris-Benedict Formula

If you ARE interested in calculating your own specific calorie numbers, you can use the Harris-Benedict Formula to determine your basal metabolic rate (BMR).

The BMR is the number of calories your body burns in a day just to keep everything functioning. To get your maintenance level, you multiply your BMR by a factor determined by your activity level. The higher your activity level, the higher your maintenance level.

Keep in mind, these are general estimates and guidelines, not "set in stone" rules! What your body requires may be far different than what's listed in a table or in a formula! When in doubt, go by your results.

If you are not gaining muscle, it's safe to say you're not eating enough calories. Raise your intake at that point by adding 200 to 300 calories to your daily total. You may need to go even higher. Your body will tell you.

Here's the formula:

1 inch = 2.54 cm
(multiply your height in inches by
2.54 to get your height in centimeters.)

1 kg = 2.2 lbs
(divide your weight in pounds by
2.2 to get your weight in kilograms)

Men:

66 + (13.7 x weight in kilograms)
+
(5 x height in centimeters)
-
(6.8 x age in years) = BMR

Women:

$$655 + (9.6 \; x \; weight \; in \; kilograms)$$
$$+$$
$$(\;1.8 \; x \; height \; in \; centimeters)$$
$$-$$
$$(4.7 \; x \; age \; in \; years) = BMR$$

To find your maintenance level, multiply your BMR by your Activity Factor. I have used a factor of 1.55 in the tables above so as not to overestimate caloric requirements. Here's a table for determining your Activity Factor level. The resulting number will be your maintenance value. This is a general number. Take it as a guide, not a rule. Subtract 300 to 500 calories from this number to get your daily caloric intake range when on the diet phase. Add 300 to 500 calories to this number when on the "feeding" phase.

Sedentary	BMR x 1.2	Little or no exercise
Lightly Active	BMR x 1.375	Light exercise/sports 1-3 days/week
Moderately Active	BMR x 1.55	Moderate exercise/sports 3-5 days/week
Very Active	BMR x 1.725	Hard exercise/sports 6-7 days/week
Extremely Active	BMR x 1.9	Hard daily exercise/sports, and physical job, 2x per day training, marathon training, etc.

References

1. The exercise-induced growth hormone response in athletes. *Sports Med. 2003; 33(8):599-613*. Godfrey RJ, Madgwick Z, Whyte GP.

2. Catecholamine release, growth hormone secretion, and energy expenditure during exercise vs. recovery in men. *J Appl Physiol. 2000 Sep; 89(3):937-46*. Pritzlaff CJ, Wideman L, Blumer J, Jensen M, Abbott RD, Gaesser GA, Veldhuis JD, Weltman A.

3. The effect of low-carbohydrate diet on the pattern of hormonal changes during incremental, graded exercise in young men. *Int J Sport Nutr Exerc Metab. 2001 Jun; 11(2):248-57*. Langfort JL, Zarzeczny R, Nazar K, Kaciuba-Uscilko H.

4. The influence of muscle action on the acute growth hormone response to resistance exercise and short-term detraining. *Growth Horm IGF Res. 2001 Apr; 11(2):75-83*. Kraemer WJ, Dudley GA, Tesch PA, Gordon SE, Hather BM, Volek JS, Ratamess NA.

5. The time course of the human growth hormone response to a 6 s and a 30 s cycle ergometer sprint. *J Sports Sci. 2002 Jun; 20(6):487-94*. Stokes KA, Nevill ME, Hall GM, Lakomy HK.

6. Effects of resistance exercise volume and nutritional supplementation on anabolic and catabolic hormones. *Eur J Appl Physiol. 2002 Feb; 86(4):315-21.* Williams AG, Ismail AN, Sharma A, Jones DA.

7. Impact of acute exercise intensity on pulsatile growth hormone release in men. *J Appl Physiol. 1999 Aug; 87(2):498-504.* Pritzlaff CJ, Wideman L, Weltman JY, Abbott RD, Gutgesell ME, Hartman ML, Veldhuis JD, Weltman A.

8. Hormonal responses of multi-set vs. single-set heavy-resistance exercise protocols. *Can J Appl Physiol. 1997 Jun; 22(3):244-55.* Gotshalk LA, Loebel CC, Nindl BC, Putukian M, Sebastianelli WJ, Newton RU, Hakkinen K, Kraemer WJ.

9. Effect of acid-base balance on the growth hormone response to acute high-intensity cycle exercise. *J Appl Physiol. 1994 Feb; 76(2):821-9.* Gordon SE, Kraemer WJ, Vos NH, Lynch JM, Knuttgen HG.

10. Acute effects of high fat and high glucose meals on the growth hormone response to exercise. *J Clin Endocrinol Metab. 1993 Jun; 76(6):1418-22.* Cappon JP, Ipp E, Brasel JA, Cooper DM.

11. Effect of low and high intensity exercise on circulating growth hormone in men. *J Clin Endocrinol Metab. 1992 Jul; 75(1):157-62.* Felsing NE, Brasel JA, Cooper DM.

12. Endogenous anabolic hormonal and growth factor responses to heavy resistance exercise in males and females. *Int J Sports Med. 1991 Apr; 12(2):228-35.* Kraemer WJ, Gordon SE, Fleck SJ, Marchitelli LJ, Mello R, Dziados JE, Friedl K, Harman E, Maresh C, Fry AC.

13. Growth hormone responses during intermittent weightlifting exercise in men. *Eur J Appl Physiol Occup Physiol. 1984; 53(1):31-4.* Vanhelder WP, Radomski MW, Goode RC.

14. Effect of anaerobic and aerobic exercise of equal duration and work expenditure on plasma growth hormone levels. *Eur J Appl Physiol Occup Physiol. 1984; 52(3):255-7.* Vanhelder WP, Goode RC, Radomski MW.

15. Rapid carbohydrate loading after a short bout of near maximal-intensity exercise. *Med Sci Sports Exerc. 2002 Jun; 34(6):980-6.* Fairchild TJ, Fletcher S, Steele P, Goodman C, Dawson B, Fournier PA.

16. Persistence of supercompensated muscle glycogen in trained subjects after carbohydrate loading. *J Appl*

Physiol. 1997 Jan; 82(1):342-7. Goforth HW Jr, Arnall DA, Bennett BL, Law PG.

17. A carbohydrate loading regimen improves high intensity, short duration exercise performance. *Int J Sport Nutr. 1995 Jun; 5(2):110-6.* Pizza FX, Flynn MG, Duscha BD, Holden J, Kubitz ER.

18. Effect of high-intensity training on capillarization and presence of angiogenic factors in human skeletal muscle. *J Physiol. 2004 June 1; 557(Pt 2): 571–582.* Jensen L, Bangsbo J, Hellsten Y.

19. Recovery from short-term intense exercise: Its relation to capillary supply and blood lactate concentration. *Eur J Appl Physiol Occup Physiol. 1983; 52(1):98-103.* Tesch PA, Wright JE.

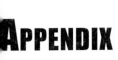

APPENDIX

Muscle Explosion Workout Sheet: Day 1

Fat Loss Circuit Training   www.sportsworkout.com/muscleexplosioncharts

Bodypart	Exercise	Sets	Reps	Notes
Chest	Dumbell Bench Press - bench or ball	3	10-6	Use a controlled movement, squeezing the pecs hard as you come to the top. Make sure you're getting good tension on the muscles and not just pushing the weight up and down.
Back	Two Dumbell Bent- Over Rows or Seated Cable Rows or Barbell Bent-Over Rows	3	10-6	With rowing exercises, don't bob your torso up and down - keep it rock steady. If you break form, lighten up the weight.
Thighs	Leg Press, Dumbbell Split Squats, or Squats (if you can pre-set bar easily)	3	10-6	Dumbell Split Squats are the easiest exercise to set up. Only to squats if you're able to pre-set the bar before you start - it just takes too much time to do setup when you're trying to keep moving through the workout.
Shoulders	Military Presses, Dumbbell Presses, or Machine Shoulder Presses	2	10-6	Dumbell presses are the best choice here - easy setup. When pressing, keep dumbells tilted down and in, like you're pouring water on your head.
Hamstrings	Leg Curls or Stiff-Legged Deadlifts	2	7-5	Hamstrings respond better to lower reps so be sure to stay on the heavy side.
Biceps	Standing Barbell Curls or Dumbbell Curls	2	10-6	Stick with the basic, heavy exercises here - no concentration curls.
Triceps	Dips, Pushdowns, or Lying Dumbbell Extensions	2	10-6	Pushdowns are a good choice - dips are good, but can be tough to get good sets at this point in the workout.
Calves	Standing or Seated Calf Raises	2	12-10	Use a controlled movement - no bouncing up and down.
	Core Combo	7	-	3 sets of abs - 2 sets of lower back - 2 sets rotator cuff

Cardiovascular Training

Activity				Comments
Fat Loss Circuit Training				Take no rest as you move between 40 seconds of cardio work and your weight training sets. Have everything set up and ready to go with your exercises as much as possible. If you are in a crowded gym and must wait for equipment or are unable to pre-set, just do the best you can.
Alternative				
Near-Maximal Aerobic Interval Training				If you are unable to adequately perform Fat Loss Circuit Training in your gym, you can substitute the Near-Maximal Aerobic Interval Training style. Do this immediately following your weight sets for 6 minutes using a "20 seconds work to 5 seconds rest" interval. Take 40 seconds rest in between all weight sets.

General Comments:

These sets are all done with a "normal" style of training. For this day, we're keeping it straightforward.

• Rep range are listed backwards (e.g. 10-6 because you should aim for 10 reps on your first set and a minimum of about 6 on your last set).

• This workout is done using the Fat Loss Circuit Training method (instructions above). If you can't use that method, do the alternative cardio as listed below it.

• When two or more exercises are listed here, select just one and do all your sets with it.

• Pre-set as many of the exercises as you can before you start to make best use of your time. In a crowded gym, this won't be practical. If you're in a crowded gym, have alternate exercises in your head that you can use if the one you want is not available. Dumbells, machines and bodyweight exercises are useful here. Barbells involve greater set-up time.

Muscle Explosion - Workout Sheet - Day 2

Fat Loss Circuit Training   www.sportsworkout.com/muscleexplosioncharts

Bodypart	Exercise	Sets	Reps	Notes
Chest	Flat Barbell or Incline Dumbell Bench Press	4	12-6	Barbell bench is preferred here - if you can't, then use incline dumbell press for variety from the previous workout.
Back	Chin-Ups, Pulldowns or Barbell Bent-Over Rows	4	12-6	The barbell row is a good one here because you'll generally be able to use the same weight as you did for the barbell bench press.
Thighs	Leg Press, Dumbell Split Squats, Squats (if you are able to pre-set the bar easily)	4	12-6	I like Leg Press for this exercise - no balance required, which is a good thing at this point in the training.
Shoulders	Military Press or Dumbell Presses or Machine Shoulder Presses	3	12-6	Remember to keep your core tight when pressing.
Hamstrings	Leg Curls or Stiff-Legged Deadlifts (barbell or dumbell)	3	7-5	Dumbell Stiff-Legged Deadlifts work well here - quick set-up.
Biceps	Standing Barbell Curls, Dumbell Curls or Cable Curls	3	12- 6	Start with a lighter weight than you think you'll need - the biceps will tire fairly quickly at this point.
Triceps	Dips, Pushdowns or Lying Dumbell Extensions	3	12-6	Lying dumbell extensions work well here.
Calves	Standing or Seated Calf Raises	3	15-10	Do whichever exercise you didn't do yesterday.
	Core Combo	7	-	3 sets of abs - 2 sets of lower back - 2 sets rotator cuff

Cardiovascular Training

Activity				Comments
Fat Loss Circuit Training				Take no rest as you move between 20 seconds of cardio work and your weight training sets. Use a higher resistance level/speed because of the shorter cardio. Have everything set up and ready to go with your exercises as much as possible. If you are in a crowded gym and must wait for equipment or are unable to pre-set, just do the best you can.
Alternative				
Near-Maximal Aerobic Interval Training				If you are unable to adequately perform Fat Loss Circuit Training in your gym, you can substitute the Near-Maximal Aerobic Interval Training style. Do this immediately following your weight sets for 6 minutes using a "20 seconds work to 5 seconds rest" interval. Take 30 seconds rest in between all weight sets.

General Comments:

These sets are all done with a "normal" style of training. For this day, we're keeping it straightforward. Use moderate weights and STRICT form here.

• Today you'll be taking just 20 seconds cardio between sets and adding in sets. Because it's a shorter cardio interval, use a higher resistance level/speed.

• You'll notice the rep differential is larger here - go for 12 reps on the first set. But because you just trained all the muscles the day before, your endurance will be less and you won't be able to get as many reps as you go through the sets.

• This workout is done using the Fat Loss Circuit Training method (instructions above). If you can't use that method, do the alternative cardio as listed below it.

• When two or more exercises are listed here, select just one and do all your sets with it.

• Pre-set as many of the exercises as you can before you start to make best use of your time. In a crowded gym, this won't be practical. If you're in a crowded gym, have alternate exercises in your head that you can use if the one you want is not available. Dumbells, machines and bodyweight exercises are useful here. Barbells involve greater set-up time.

Muscle Explosion - Workout Sheet - Day 3 - Rest Day. Carb Up!

High Rep Partial Training—Lactic Acid Training Style   www.sportsworkout.com/muscleexplosioncharts

Bodypart	Exercise	Sets	Reps	Notes
Chest	Flat Barbell Bench Press Dumbell Flyes - Ball or Bench	8+2	20-30+	With the bench press, only the top lockout range. Use the rack for this. With flyes, do reps in the bottom few inches of the range. The ball works best for this rather than the bench because you can really wrap your back around it. To increase pec activation, grip the dumbells HARD.
Back	Seated Cable Rows or Barbell Bent-Over Rows Stiff-Arm ushdowns	8+2	20-30+	With the rows, only the top contracted position. Stiff-Arm Pushdowns are done on the high pulley. Lock your arms stiff and almost straight, take a step back, lean forward then push bar down in front of you. Expand your lungs and chest as much as possible on the stretch. Use only the top few inches here.
Biceps	Standing Barbell Curls Incline Dumbell Curls	6+2	20-30+	Do the standing barbell curls in the rack with the rails set high or curl the first rep up to the start position. On incline curls, puff your chest and really let the dumbells pull your arms back. Turn your palms OUT in that stretch position to maximize it. Letting them turn in takes the stretch off.
Calves	BSeated Calf Raises or Standing Calf Raises Donkey or Leg Press Calf Raises	6+2	20-30+	With standing calf raises, just the top little bit of the movement. Contract hard and squeeze, let down a little then contract hard and squeeze. Keep lower back arched with donkeys - don't round it or it'll reduce the stretch. Same on leg press.
Traps	Barbell or Dumbbell Shrugs	2	20-30+	Just 2 high rep sets here. Use a moderate weight and burn out with as many reps as your traps and grip can handle.

Cardiovascular Training - None

General Comments:

- With today's training, we really shake up the muscles in their most extreme positions. The first exercise is done in the CONTRACTED position of the range of motion. But here's the catch—that contracted position exercise should be an exercise where you can use a LOT of weight. Example: Even though concentration curls are a more contracted position, we'll use the barbell curl because you can go much heavier.

- Because this is Lactic Acid Training, use a light to moderate weight and do as many reps as you can on the first set (you will get fewer reps on successive sets). That means you should get the 20 to 30+ reps ONLY on the first set. If you can still get those reps on the next sets, you're not using enough eight.

- Rest 20 seconds. Then go immediately to the OTHER exercise, which will focus on the STRETCH position of the muscle. The range is short; do only the bottom few inches of the STRETCH position.

- Alternate the two exercises for the number of sets on the left. Example: 8 sets for chest will look like flyes, press, flyes, press, flyes, press, flyes, press. It's 4 sets of each exercise.

- Be sure you're using a VERY DELIBERATE stretch and contraction on the exercises. THAT is where the real benefit of this technique lies.

- When you get to the "+2" sets, those are going to be two VERY high rep set (40 to 50+ reps!) of the contracted position exercise, e.g. bench press. Use a FULL range of motion and very light weight. Go for as many reps as you can do and feel the burn! Rest 1 minute before you start this high-rep set on each bodypart and rest 1 minute between the two sets.

Muscle Explosion - Workout Sheet - Day 5

High Rep Partial Training - Lactic Acid Training Style www.sportsworkout.com/muscleexplosioncharts

Bodypart	Exercise	Sets	Reps	Notes
Shoulders	Barbell, Dumbell or Machine Shoulder Press Barbell, Dumbell or Machine Shoulder Press	6+2	20-30+	Shoulders are tough to get a good stretch on so I've gone with the bottom of the pressing movement (any apparatus). Just focus on keeping the tension on at the bottom - no resting the bar on the upper chest. Use the rack to do top range barbell presses - I like to alternate kneeling barbell press (top range) then stand up with the same rack height and do bottom range shoulder press. If you're doing Dumbell Presses for the bottom, use the W press (palms facing in towards your head). To get the best stretch, hold the dumbells up near the base of your fingers, then let your hands bend backwards. It will feel like you're a waiter carrying a drink tray. This puts more stretch on the delts.
Triceps	Weighted Dips or Close Grip Bench Press Bodyweight Tricep Extensions or Overhead Dumbell or Barbell Ext. or Overhead Cable Extensions	6+2	20-30+	Weighted dips are great for the top range exercise - you can do these in the rack with two barbells set across the safety rails to use as dipping bars. Close grip bench is good, too - just keep your elbows close to your body. The stretch exercise for triceps can put some stress on your elbows so be very careful and deliberate with this one - no bouncing.
Hamstrings	Leg Curls Stiff-Legged Deadlifts	6+2	20-30+	For leg curls, only do the top few inches. Contract hard! Use leg curls for the full range, high-rep exercise. When doing Stiff Legged Deadlifts, elevate your toes on a plate or foam wedges to increase stretch on hams. Just do the bottom few inches and keep in the stretch. Another good trick is to use small plates (25's) so that you increase the range of motion on the stretch. Stretch as far as you can WITHOUT rounding the lower back. If your lower back starts to lose the arch, you've gone too far.
Thighs	Top 1/4 Squats - no lockout Sissy Squats or Bottom Leg Press	8+2	20-30+	With the 1/4 squats, DO NOT go to lockout. That will take tension off the quads. Stop just short then go back down. Do light, full-range squats for the +2 exercise. Sissy squats are the preferred exercise here as they provide the greatest stretch. If your knees can't take Sissy Squats, do just the bottom few inches of the Leg Press. I like to do Sissy Squats in the rack, holding onto the safety rails to help spot and balance for maximum stretch.
Traps	Shrugs, Barbell or Dumbbell	2	20-30+	Just 2 high rep sets here. Use a moderate weight and burn out with as many reps as you traps and grip can handle. No pausing at the bottom, just a very quick movement.

Cardiovascular Training - None

General Comments:

- With todays training, we're going to really shake up the muscles in their most extreme positions. The first exercise is done in the CONTRACTED position of the range of motion. But here's the catch - that contracted position exercise should be an exercises where you can use a LOT of weight, e.g. even though concentration curls are a more contracted position, we'll use the barbell curl because you can go much heavier.

- Because this is Lactic Acid Training, use a light to moderate weight and do as many reps as you can on the first set (you will get fewer reps on successive sets). That means you should get the 20 to 30+ reps ONLY on the first set. If you can still get those reps on the next sets, you're not using enough weight.

- Rest 20 seconds. Then go immediately to the OTHER exercise, which will focus on the STRETCH position of the muscle. The range is short, doing only the bottom few inches of the STRETCH position.

- Alternate those two exercises for the number of sets on the left (e.g. 8 sets for chest will look like flyes, press, flyes, press, flyes, press, flyes, press) It'll be 4 sets of each exercise.

- Be sure you're using a VERY DELIBERATE stretch and contraction on the exercises. THAT is where the real benefit of this technique lies.

- When you get to the "+2" sets, those are going to be two VERY high rep set (40 to 50+ reps!) of the contracted position exercise, e.g. bench press. Use a FULL range of motion and very light weight. Go for as many reps as you can do and feel the burn! Rest 1 minute before you start this high-rep set on each bodypart and rest 1 minute between the two sets..

Muscle Explosion - Workout Sheet - Day 6

Interval Training + Core Combo   www.sportsworkout.com/muscleexplosioncharts

BODYPART	EXERCISE	SETS	REPS	NOTES
Abs	Curl Squats	2	4-6	This is a great exercise for building support strength in the abs. Start with a moderate weight so you get an idea of how much you can use. It's a very tough one!
Abs	Two Dumbell Ball Twists or Cable-Gripping Trunk Twists	2	4-6	This exercise should be a rotational-based exercise. It'll help tighten up the core.
Lower Back	Hyperextensions	2	6-8	Do these under control - hold at the top and squeeze.
Rotator Cuff	3 in 1 Rotator Cuff Exercise	2	6-10	Choose either one of these exercises. Working the Rotator Cuff helps tremendously with shoulder stability.

Cardiovascular Training

Activity	Comments
15 minutes Sub-Maximal Interval Training	30 seconds at about 80- 90% then 30 seconds slow for 15 minutes. We're NOT pushing to the limit here. It should be hard work but not blasting hard. We're just trying to raise the metabolism and get some blood flowing but without seriously impairing overall recovery.

General Comments:

- Today, start with Sub-maximal interval training first. Then you'll go to the Core Combo, with the ab exercises, lower back and rotator cuff following that.

- With the interval training, DO NOT push yourself as hard as you can. It should be somewhat hard but we're not trying to destroy you here - just get some reasonably intense cardio.

- This will help you with recovery while not slowing down muscle growth by going too intense.

Muscle Explosion - Workout Sheet - Day 7 - Rest Day.

Technique	Exercise	Sets x Reps	Notes
20 minutes of Compound Exercise Overload on Target Exercise	Deadlifts or Squats or Other Exercise	Sets of 3 reps for 20 minutes - 30 seconds rest between sets REST 2 MINUTES then do 1 set of as many reps as you can do with the last weight you used.	If this is your first time through the program, do deadlifts or squats, NOT any other exercise. We need to work on either of the two exercises that are going to do the most for overall mass building. Those are squats and deadlifts. When you do a second round of the program, THEN you can try a different exercise. If ARE doing a different exercise, take only 20 SECONDS rest between sets. Squats and deadlifts, being more overall demanding than most exercises go better with a little more rest. Also, when doing squats and deadlifts, drop the weight 20 lbs on weight changes instead of 10 with other exercises. If you can't keep TIGHT form on ANY rep of any set, REDUCE THE WEIGHT. This is a critical point. Any technique errors will be amplified by the high volume of training.

WRITE YOUR STARTING WEIGHT AND ENDING WEIGHT HERE

Start Weight:		Time Used For:	
End Weight		Time Used For:	

General Comments:

- The training today is very challenging and is only just the first day! Basically, start with a weight you can do for 6 reps and do 3 reps with it. Rest 30 seconds then do another set of 3 reps with it. Keep going until you can't do 3 reps. Drop the weight 20 pounds (for squats and deadlifts - 10 lbs for other exercises) then go again with the 3 rep sets. Repeat this for 20 minutes.

- DO NOT go to failure on ANY of your sets! The idea here is to to overload the body with training volume, not intensity.

- Stick with 3 reps - your body hits a rep-range groove and will acclimate to it very quickly. Keeps your nervous system efficient.

- If you're REALLY suffering and can't keep up even with weight changes, take a full minute rest to try and recover a bit. Then keep going.

- On the final set (after 20 minutes are up) rest for TWO FULL minutes then get as many reps as you can with the same weight.

- The training uses neuromuscular specificity to allow you to teach your body the absolute most efficient way to perform a single exercise. Your body will learn to fire the exact sequence of muscles it needs to do the exercise, making fast strength gains possible.

- Don't use different variations of the same exercise. It's important to use the EXACT SAME exercise the whole 20 mintues.

- Do your best with the 30 second rest - this will increase a bit during weight changes.

- This technique will give you a deep engorgement of blood to your target muscles.

- Keep track of your starting weight and ending weight so you know what to improve on with the next training day (tomorrow!). Our goal is going to be to increase the starting weight each for at least the first 3 days of this week-long cycle.

- When you do this exercise with squats, try to increase your range of motion as you lighten the weight - oftentimes, the tendency with heavy weights is to shorten the range of motion, which is fine. Just try to go deeper as you get lighter.

Technique	Exercise	Sets x Reps	Notes
25 minutes of Compound Exercise Overload on Target Exercise	Deadlifts or Squats	Sets of 3 reps for 25 minutes - 30 seconds rest between sets REST 2 MINUTES then do 1 set of as many reps as you can do with the last weight you used.	Today, increase the weight a bit for your first set. Even though you just trained hard yesterday, your nervous system will be better tuned to the exercise and you'll probably be a bit stronger at it! Remember, 30 seconds rest if you're doing squats or deadlifts - 20 seconds with any other exercise.

WRITE YOUR STARTING WEIGHT AND ENDING WEIGHT HERE

Start Weight:		Time Used For:	
End Weight		Time Used For:	

General Comments:

- Start with a weight you can do for 6 reps and do 3 reps with it. Rest 30 seconds then do another set of 3 reps with it. Keep going until you can't do 3 reps. Drop the weight 10 pounds then go again with the 3 rep sets. Repeat this for 25 minutes.

- DO NOT go to failure on ANY of your sets! The idea here is to to overload the body with training volume, not intensity.

- On the final set (after 25 minutes are up) rest for a 2 FULL minutes then get as many reps as you can with the same weight.

- Don't use different variations of the same exercise. It's important to use the EXACT SAME exercise the whole 25 mintues.

- Do your best with the 30 second rest - this may increase a bit during weight changes.

- Keep track of your starting weight and ending weight so you know what to improve on with the next training day (tomorrow!). Our goal is going to be to increase the starting weight each for at least the first 3 days of this week-long cycle.

- Expect a faster drop in weight today as your muscles will probably be sore and you won't be able to hold the same strength levels for as long as the previous day.

Muscle Explosion - Workout Sheet - Day 10

Compound Exercise Overload Day 3   www.sportsworkout.com/muscleexplosioncharts

Technique	Exercise	Sets x Reps	Notes
30 minutes of Compound Exercise Overload on Target Exercise	Deadlifts or Squats	Sets of 3 reps for 30 minutes - 30 seconds rest between sets REST 2 MINUTES then do 1 set of as many reps as you can do with the last weight you used.	Again, try to increase the weight on your starting sets. We're trying to force adaptation by steadily increasing the load on the body. This is going to be a tough workout as the workload will start to really catch up to you today.

WRITE YOUR STARTING WEIGHT AND ENDING WEIGHT HERE			
Start Weight:		Time Used For:	
End Weight		Time Used For:	

General Comments:

- Start with a weight you can do for 6 reps and do 3 reps with it. Rest 30 seconds then do another set of 3 reps with it. Keep going until you can't do 3 reps. Drop the weight 20 pounds (10 for other exercises than squats and deadlifts) then go again with the 3 rep sets. Repeat this for 30 minutes.

- DO NOT go to failure on ANY of your sets! The idea here is to to overload the body with training volume, not intensity.

- On the final set (after 30 minutes are up) rest for TWO FULL minutes then get as many reps as you can with the same weight.

- Don't use different variations of the same exercise. It's important to use the EXACT SAME exercise the whole 30 mintues.

- Do your best with the 30 second rest - this will increase a bit during weight changes.

- Keep track of your starting weight and ending weight so you know what to improve on with the next training day (tomorrow!). Our goal is going to be to increase the starting weight each for at least the first 3 days of this week-long cycle.

Muscle Explosion - Workout Sheet - Day 10 - Adapted

Compound Exercise Overload Day 3   www.sportsworkout.com/muscleexplosioncharts

Technique	Exercise	Sets x Reps	Notes
25 minutes of Compound Exercise Overload on Target Exercise	Deadlifts or Squats	Sets of 3 reps for 25 minutes - 30 seconds rest between sets REST 2 MINUTES then do 1 set of as many reps as you can do with the last weight you used.	Again, try to increase the weight on your starting sets. We're trying to force adaptation by steadily increasing the load on the body. This is going to be a tough workout as the workload will start to really catch up to you today.

WRITE YOUR STARTING WEIGHT AND ENDING WEIGHT HERE			
Start Weight:		Time Used For:	
End Weight		Time Used For:	

General Comments:

- Start with a weight you can do for 6 reps and do 3 reps with it. Rest 30 seconds then do another set of 3 reps with it. Keep going until you can't do 3 reps. Drop the weight 20 pounds (10 for other exercises than squats and deadlifts) then go again with the 3 rep sets. Repeat this for 25 minutes.

- DO NOT go to failure on ANY of your sets! The idea here is to to overload the body with training volume, not intensity.

- On the final set (after 25 minutes are up) rest for TWO FULL minutes then get as many reps as you can with the same weight.

- Don't use different variations of the same exercise. It's important to use the EXACT SAME exercise the whole 25 mintues.

- Do your best with the 30 second rest - this will increase a bit during weight changes.

- Keep track of your starting weight and ending weight so you know what to improve on with the next training day (after a day or rest tomorrow).

Compound Exercise Overload Day 4   www.sportsworkout.com/muscleexplosioncharts

Technique	Exercise	Sets x Reps	Notes
35 minutes of Compound Exercise Overload on Target Exercise	Deadlifts or Squats	Sets of 3 reps for 30 minutes - 30 seconds rest between sets REST 2 MINUTES then do 1 set of as many reps as you can do with the last weight you used.	If you feel like you can, increase your starting weight again. But if you don't feel like you've got it in you, don't. The constant workload is catching up to you and the body is going to go into emergency mode. You're really digging into the reserves here. In my experience, even when you can start heavier, once you have to drop weight, you will start dropping the weight FAST. The top-end strength is there but the volume-endurance is down a lot.

WRITE YOUR STARTING WEIGHT AND ENDING WEIGHT HERE

Start Weight:		Time Used For:	
End Weight		Time Used For:	

General Comments:

- Start with a weight you can do for 6 reps and do 3 reps with it. Rest 30 seconds then do another set of 3 reps with it. Keep going until you can't do 3 reps. Drop the weight 20 pounds then go again with the 3 rep sets. Repeat this for 35 minutes.

- DO NOT go to failure on ANY of your sets! The idea here is to to overload the body with training volume, not intensity.

- If you have to take a break anywhere in the course of the workout (and that is fine!), stop the timer so the clock isn't still ticking on the workout. Take a couple of minutes to get a bit better recovery, then go again and restart the timer.

- On the final set (after 35 minutes are up) rest for TWO FULL minutes then get as many reps as you can with the same weight.

- Don't use different variations of the same exercise. It's important to use the EXACT SAME exercise the whole 35 mintues.

- Do your best with the 30 second rest - this will increase a bit during weight changes.

- Keep track of your starting weight and ending weight.

Muscle Explosion - Workout Sheet - Day 12

Compound Exercise Overload Day 5   www.sportsworkout.com/muscleexplosioncharts

Technique	Exercise	Sets x Reps	Notes
40 minutes of Compound Exercise Overload on Target Exercise	Deadlifts or Squats	Sets of 3 reps for 30 minutes - 30 seconds rest between sets REST 2 MINUTES then do 1 set of as many reps as you can do with the last weight you used.	On this final day, you may need to reduce the starting weight so that you can actually get reps here. I recommend going back to the ORIGINAL weight that you did on the first day of this training style. It's the toughest day because your body will be going on fumes. It's fine to reduce the weight so that you can keep good form and perform the full 40 minute workout. When doing squats or deadlifts, drop the weight 30 lbs on each drop today. If you're doing any other exercise, drop 20 lbs instead of 10. Trust me on this. You'll need the increased weight drop.

WRITE YOUR STARTING WEIGHT AND ENDING WEIGHT HERE

Start Weight:		Time Used For:	
End Weight		Time Used For:	

General Comments:

- Start with a weight you can do for 6 reps and do 3 reps with it. Rest 30 seconds then do another set of 3 reps with it. Keep going until you can't do 3 reps. Drop the weight 30 pounds then go again with the 3 rep sets. Repeat this for 40 minutes.

- DO NOT go to failure on ANY of your sets! The idea here is to to overload the body with training volume, not intensity.

- On the final set (after 40 minutes are up) rest for TWO FULL minutes then get as many reps as you can with the same weight.

- Don't use different variations of the same exercise. It's important to use the EXACT SAME exercise the whole 40 mintues.

- Do your best with the 30 second rest - this will increase a bit during weight changes.

- Keep track of your starting weight and ending weight.

Muscle Explosion - Workout Sheet - Day 12 - Adapted

Compound Exercise Overload Day 5   www.sportsworkout.com/muscleexplosioncharts

Technique	Exercise	Sets x Reps	Notes
30 minutes of Compound Exercise Overload on Target Exercise	Deadlifts or Squats	Sets of 3 reps for 30 minutes - 30 seconds rest between sets REST 2 MINUTES then do 1 set of as many reps as you can do with the last weight you used	On this final day, you may need to reduce the starting weight so that you can actually get reps here. I recommend going back to the ORIGINAL weight that you did on the first day of this training style. It's the toughest day because your body will be going on fumes. It's fine to reduce the weight so that you can keep good form and perform the full 30 minute workout. When doing squats or deadlifts, drop the weight 30 lbs on each drop today. If you're doing any other exercise, drop 20 lbs instead of 10. Trust me on this. You'll need the increased weight drop.

WRITE YOUR STARTING WEIGHT AND ENDING WEIGHT HERE

Start Weight:		Time Used For:	
End Weight		Time Used For:	

General Comments:

- Start with a weight you can do for 6 reps and do 3 reps with it. Rest 30 seconds then do another set of 3 reps with it. Keep going until you can't do 3 reps. Drop the weight 30 pounds then go again with the 3 rep sets. Repeat this for 30 minutes.

- DO NOT go to failure on ANY of your sets! The idea here is to to overload the body with training volume, not intensity.

- On the final set (after 30 minutes are up) rest for TWO FULL minutes then get as many reps as you can with the same weight.

- Don't use different variations of the same exercise. It's important to use the EXACT SAME exercise the whole 30 mintues.

- Do your best with the 30 second rest - this will increase a bit during weight changes.

- Keep track of your starting weight and ending weight.

Muscle Explosion - Workout Sheet - Day 13 & 14 - Rest Days

Stretch-Pause Training www.sportsworkout.com/muscleexplosioncharts

Bodypart	Exercise	Sets	Reps	Notes
Chest	Flat Barbell Bench Press and Dumbell Flyes	3	10, ?, ?	No bouncing on the bench press to get more reps. These should be done under control and squeezing the chest to make sure you get the reps. To maximize tension on the last rep of the last set, you can do a static hold at the top for as long as you can.
Back	Barbell Rows or Cable Rows and Stiff-Arm Pushdowns or Dumbell Pullovers	3	10, ?, ?	I like to do barbell rows and use the same weight as I just used for bench press. It makes it easier to set up. Do pullovers on the Swiss Ball to get the best stretch.
Biceps	Standing Dumbell or Barbell Curls and Incline Curls	2	10, ?, ?	With curls, go lighter than you think you'll need to so that you can keep tight form and still get the reps. If you go too heavy, it's too easy to cheat and lose tension.
Calves	Standing or Seated Calf Raises and Donkey Calf Raises or Leg Press Calf Raises	2	10, ?, ?	Get a good stretch at the bottom of each rep. When you come up to the top of each rep, try to focus on coming up on the big toe knuckles on the balls of your feet - better overall calf contraction.
Traps	Dumbell Shrugs or Dumbell Farmers Walk	4	10, ?, ?	Just do one rest-pause set with the heaviest dumbells you have access to or can handle for 10 reps. Dumbells are shorter in terms of set-up time. Look up at about a 45 degree angle and keep your chest puffed out and shoulders back. This will help activate the traps. To do a Farmer's Walk, you just hold 2 heavy dumbells then walk as far as you can with them.
	Abbreviated Core Combo		-	1 set of abs - 1 set of lower back - 2 sets rotator cuff

Cardiovascular Training - None

General Comments:

• Today is Stretch-Pause Training, meaning on your first set, use a weight that you can get 10 reps with. Do the 10, Stretch 20 seconds, then do the OTHER exercise (a stretch-accentuated exercise with a full range of motion), holding the stretch for 3 to 5 seconds on each rep) for as many MORE reps as you can (probably around 4 to 6). Stretch 20 seconds, then finish with as many more reps as you can get on the FIRST exercise again, using only the top, partial range of motion.

• On the stretch exercise, use a weight you could normally get about 12 to 15 reps with.

• As an example, this would look like 10 reps bench press, 6 reps dumbell flyes, 3 reps bench press.

• This layout is the reason for the "?" in the reps column above. Since I don't know how many reps you'll get, I didn't state a rep target - just as many as possible!

• One "set" in this workout means one time through the three mini-sets. THEN you would take your 90 seconds rest in between those Stretch-Pause sets.

• If you can, set up your next exercise during the rest period between Stretch-Pause sets. This will help you keep things moving between exercises.

• It's critical that you go for TENSION in the muscles in these sets. Don't just blast out reps. Do them under control and really squeeze the muscles. This will get you best results.

• Write down the weights you use for each exercise so you can track progress and add weight next time you use that exercise again.

• NOTE: on this day, you may find your starting weights aren't what you expect - you may not have recovered quite enough from the previous week's training, especially if you did squats or dead lifts.

Stretch-Pause Training   www.sportsworkout.com/muscleexplosioncharts

Bodypart	Exercise	Sets	Reps	Notes
Shoulders	Barbell, Dumbell or Machine Shoulder Press	2	10, ?, ?	Any form of pressing will be fine here. Best to go with a version that you didn't use on Day 16. With shoulders, we're not doing any stretch-pause sets, only straight rest-pause training. There aren't any REALLY good stretch-position exercises for the shoulders and you'll get a better mass-building effect with the presses. When choosing which type of press to use, be sure to rotate, e.g. do barbells today then dumbells the next time.
Triceps	Close Grip Bench Press and Lying Tricep Extensions (or overhead)	2	10, ?, ?	You can use either variation of the tricep extension as long as you get a good stretch on the triceps.
Thighs	No Squats - Use Split Squats, Lunges, or Leg Press and Sissy Squats	3	10, ?, ?	The reason for no squats today is that if you did squats or deadlifts for the 5 day Attack last week, your legs will still be trashed (trust me). If you were an upper body exercise during the 5 days, you CAN do squats today.
Hamstrings	Leg Curls and Stiff-Legged Dead lifts	2	6, ?, ?	Since hamstrings respond better to low reps, aim for 6 on the first set.
Traps	Dumbell Shrugs or Dumbell Farmers Walk	1	10, ?, ?	Just do one rest-pause set with the heaviest dumbells you have access to or can handle for 10 reps. Dumbells are shorter in terms of set-up time. Look up at about a 45 degree angle and keep your chest puffed out and shoulders back. This will help activate the traps. To do a Farmer's Walk, you just hold 2 heavy dumbells then walk as far as you can with them.
	Abbreviated Core Combo	4	-	1 set of abs - 1 set of lower back - 2 sets rotator cuff

Cardiovascular Training - None

General Comments:

- Today is Stretch-Pause Training, meaning on your first set, use a weight that you can get 10 reps with. Do the 10, rest 20 seconds, then do the OTHER exercise (a stretch-accentuated exercise with a full range of motion, holding the stretch for 3 to 5 seconds on each rep) for as many MORE reps as you can (probably around 4 to 6). Rest 20 seconds, then finish with as many more reps as you can get on the FIRST exercise again, using only the top, partial range of motion.

- On the stretch exercise, use a weight you could normally get about 12 to 15 reps with.

- Remember to hold the stretch position for 3 to 5 seconds on each stretch set!

- This layout is the reason for the "?" in the reps column above. Since I don't know how many reps you'll get, I didn't state a rep target - just as many as possible!

- One "set" in this workout means one time through the three mini-sets. THEN take 90 seconds rest in between those Stretch-Pause sets.

- If you can, set up your next exercise during the rest period between Stretch-Pause sets. This will help you keep things moving between exercises.

- It's critical that you go for TENSION in the muscles in these sets. Don't just blast out reps. Do them under control and really squeeze the muscles. This will get you best results.

- Write down the weights you use for each exercise so you can track progress and add weight next time you use that exercise again.

Muscle Explosion - Workout Sheet - Day 17 - Rest Day.

Muscle Explosion - Workout Sheet - Day 18

Stretch-Pause Training   www.sportsworkout.com/muscleexplosioncharts

Bodypart	Exercise	Sets	Reps	Notes
Chest	Dumbell Bench Press and Dumbell Flyes	2	10, ?, ?	Do dumbell bench press today because you did barbell on the first day of this week.
Back	Chins or Weighted Chins or Deadlifts and Stiff-Arm Pushdowns	2	10, ?, ?	With this one, do a chin-up (or weighted, if you can use extra weight for 10 reps). If you can't do 10 chin- ups, use a heavy pulldown but chins are preferred. If you did an upper body exercise for the 5 day attack, you can use Deadlifts here instead of the chinning movement. If you DO use deadlifts, do rest-pause training, using deadlifts for all 3 mini-sets - NO stretch exercise! To increase the stretch on Stiff-Arm Pushdowns, rotate the bar 90 degrees to the left or right at the top of the movement (reverse on next rep).
Biceps	Reverse Barbell Curls and Incline Curls	3	10, ?, ?	Today, we're using the underappreciated Reverse Curl to fill out the lower arm (brachialis). Like Day 15, use a lighter weight than you think you need and go for very form and high tension. That will give you best results. No fast, pumping momentum reps here
Calves	Standing or Seated Calf Raises and Donkey Calf Raises or Leg Press Calf Raises	2	10, ?, ?	Get a good stretch at the bottom of each rep. Use any exercise that you didn't use on Day 15.
Traps	Dumbell Shrugs or Dumbell Farmers Walk	1	10, ?, ?	Just do one rest-pause set with the heaviest dumbells you have access to or can handle for 10 reps. Dumbells are shorter in terms of set-up time. Look up at about a 45 degree angle and keep your chest puffed out and shoulders back. This will help activate the traps. To do a Farmer's Walk, you just hold 2 heavy dumbells then walk as far as you can with them.
	Abbreviated Core Combo	4	-	1 set of abs - 1 set of lower back - 2 sets rotator cuff

Cardiovascular Training - None

General Comments:

- Today is Stretch-Pause Training, meaning on your first set, use a weight that you can get 10 reps with. Do the 10, rest 20 seconds, then do the OTHER exercise (a stretch-accentuated exercise with a full range of motion, holding the stretch for 3 to 5 seconds on each rep) for as many MORE reps as you can (probably around 4 to 6). Rest 20 seconds, then finish with as many more reps as you can get on the FIRST exercise again, using only the top, partial range of motion.

- On the stretch exercise, use a weight you could normally get about 12 to 15 reps with.

- Remember to hold the stretch position for 3 to 5 seconds on each stretch set!

- This layout is the reason for the "?" in the reps column above. Since I don't know how many reps you'll get, I didn't state a rep target - just as many as possible!

- One "set" in this workout means one time through the three mini-sets. THEN take 90 seconds rest in between those Stretch-Pause sets.

- If you can, set up your next exercise during the rest period between Stretch-Pause sets. This will help you keep things moving between exercises.

- It's critical that you go for TENSION in the muscles in these sets. Don't just blast out reps. Do them under control and really squeeze the muscles. This will get you best results.

- Write down the weights you use for each exercise so you can track progress and add weight next time you use that exercise again.

Stretch-Pause Training   www.sportsworkout.com/muscleexplosioncharts

Bodypart	Exercise	Sets	Reps	Notes
Triceps	Decline Close Grip Presses or Dips/ Weighted Dips and Tricep Extensions	2	10, ?, ?	The decline close grip press allows you to use maximum weight for triceps. Parallel bar dips or weighted dips (if you can get 10 reps with weight) will work great here as well. We're doing triceps before shoulders because you can use more weight with close grip presses and dips than shoulder presses.
Shoulders	Barbell, Dumbell or Machine Shoulder Press	2	10, ?, ?	Any form of pressing will be fine here. Best to go with a version that you didn't use on Day 16. With shoulders, we're not doing any stretch-pause sets, only straight rest-pause training. There aren't any REALLY good stretch-position exercises for the shoulders and you'll get a better mass-building effect with the presses. When choosing which type of press to use, be sure to rotate, e.g. do barbells today then dumbells the next time.
Thighs	Dumbell Split Squats or Leg Press - Squats if you did an upper body during the 5 day attack. and Sissy Squats	3	10, ?, ?	You should be fine to do squats today IF you did an upper body exercise during the 5 day attack If you did deadlifts or squats during the 5 day, do splits squats or leg press. We'll be hitting squats hard next week!
Hamstrings	Leg Curls and Stiff-Legged Deadlifts	2	6, ?, ?	The preferred exercise is Stiff Legged Deadlifts but use Leg Curls if SLDL's hurt your lower back.
Traps	Dumbell Shrugs or Dumbell Farmers Walk	1	10, ?, ?	Just do one rest-pause set with the heaviest dumbells you have access to or can handle for 10 reps. Dumbells are shorter in terms of set-up time. Look up at about a 45 degree angle and keep your chest puffed out and shoulders back. This will help activate the traps. To do a Farmer's Walk, you just hold 2 heavy dumbells then walk as far as you can with them.
	Abbreviated Core Combo	4	-	1 set of abs - 1 set of lower back - 2 sets rotator cuff

Cardiovascular Training - None

General Comments:

- Today is Stretch-Pause Training, meaning on your first set, use a weight that you can get 10 reps with. Do the 10, rest 20 seconds, then do the OTHER exercise (a stretch-accentuated exercise with a full range of motion, holding the stretch for 3 to 5 seconds on each rep) for as many MORE reps as you can (probably around 4 to 6). Rest 20 seconds, then finish with as many more reps as you can get on the FIRST exercise again, using only the top, partial range of motion.

- On the stretch exercise, use a weight you could normally get about 12 to 15 reps with.

- Remember to hold the stretch position for 3 to 5 seconds on each stretch set!

- This layout is the reason for the "?" in the reps column above. Since I don't know how many reps you'll get, I didn't state a rep target - just as many as possible!

- One "set" in this workout means one time through the three mini-sets. THEN take 90 seconds rest in between those Stretch-Pause sets.

- If you can, set up your next exercise during the rest period between Stretch-Pause sets. This will help you keep things moving between exercises.

- It's critical that you go for TENSION in the muscles in these sets. Don't just blast out reps. Do them under control and really squeeze the muscles. This will get you best results.

- Write down the weights you use for each exercise so you can track progress and add weight next time you use that exercise again.

Muscle Explosion - Workout Sheet - Day 20 & 21 - Rest Days.

Muscle Explosion - Workout Sheet - Day 22

Stretch-Pause Training   www.sportsworkout.com/muscleexplosioncharts

Bodypart	Exercise	Sets	Reps	Notes
Back	Deadlifts	3	10, ?, ?	Use a weight that will really challenge you to get 10 reps. You'll get fewer reps on the next Rest-Pause sets but don't worry about it. Go for broke on the first set. When doing deadlifts, DO NOT do Stretch-Pause training. Because the deadlift is one of THE most effective muscle-building exercises, do a rest-pause set - 10 reps of deadlifts, rest 20 seconds, as many reps of deadlifts, rest 20 seconds, as many as you can get to finish.
Chest	Flat Barbell Bench Press or Half-Range Machine Bench Press and Dumbell Flyes	3	10, ?, ?	No bouncing on the bench press to get more reps. These should be done under control and squeezing the chest to make sure you get the reps. To maximize tension on the last rep of the last set, you can do a static hold at the top for as long as you can. Machine bench presses are fine to do here - use a half range of motion to help avoid shoulder trouble on the machines. Use a VERY controlled, tension-focused movement here, pausing at the top and the mid-point of each rep to maximize that tension.
Biceps	Standing Dumbell or Barbell Curls (EZ Bar is okay here) and Incline Curls	2	10, ?, ?	With curls, go lighter than you think you'll need to so that you can keep tight form and still get the reps. If you go heavy, it's too easy to cheat and lose tension.
Calves	Standing or Seated Calf Raises and Donkey or Leg Press Calf Raises	2	10, ?, ?	Get a good stretch at the bottom of each rep.
Traps	Dumbell Shrugs or Dumbell Farmers Walk	1	10, ?, ?	Just do one rest-pause set with the heaviest dumbells you have access to or can handle for 10 reps. Dumbells are shorter in terms of set-up time. Look up at about a 45 degree angle and keep your chest puffed out and shoulders back. This will help activate the traps. To do a Farmer's Walk, you just hold 2 heavy dumbells then walk as far as you can with them.
	Abbreviated Core Combo	4	-	1 set of abs - 1 set of lower back - 2 sets rotator cuff

Cardiovascular Training - None

General Comments:

- Today is Stretch-Pause Training, meaning on your first set, use a weight that you can get 10 reps with. Do the 10, rest 20 seconds, then do the OTHER exercise (a stretch-accentuated exercise with a full range of motion, holding the stretch for 3 to 5 seconds on each rep) for as many MORE reps as you can (probably around 4 to 6). Rest 20 seconds, then finish with as many more reps as you can get on the FIRST exercise again, using only the top, partial range of motion.

- On the stretch exercise, use a weight you could normally get about 12 to 15 reps with.

- Remember to hold the stretch position for 3 to 5 seconds on each stretch set!

- This layout is the reason for the "?" in the reps column above. Since I don't know how many reps you'll get, I didn't state a rep target - just as many as possible!

- One "set" in this workout means one time through the three mini-sets. THEN take 90 seconds rest in between those Stretch-Pause sets.

- If you can, set up your next exercise during the rest period between Stretch-Pause sets. This will help you keep things moving between exercises.

- It's critical that you go for TENSION in the muscles in these sets. Don't just blast out reps. Do them under control and really squeeze the muscles. This will get you best results.

- Write down the weights you use for each exercise so you can track progress and add weight next time you use that exercise again.

Muscle Explosion - Workout Sheet - Day 23

Stretch-Pause Training   www.sportsworkout.com/muscleexplosioncharts

Bodypart	Exercise	Sets	Reps	Notes
Shoulders	Barbell, Dumbell or Machine Shoulder Press	2	10, ?, ?	Any form of pressing will be fine here. Best to go with a version that you didn't use on Day 16. With shoulders, we're not doing any stretch-pause sets, only straight rest-pause training. There aren't any REALLY good stretch-position exercises for the shoulders and you'll get a better mass-building effect with the presses. When choosing which type of press to use, be sure to rotate, e.g. do barbells today then dumbells the next time.
Triceps	Close Grip Presses and Tricep Extensions	2	10, ?, ?	Use either overhead or lying tricep extensions.
Thighs	Squats	3	10, ?, ?	Be sure you're getting full squats here to maximize the anabolic effect of the exercise. Do straight Rest-Pause Training with the squat. No Stretch-Pause. Squats are one of the best mass-building exercises. We want to take advantage of that here. Do 10 reps, then rest 20 seconds, then do as many more squats as you can, rest 20 seconds, then finish with as many more as you can.
Hamstrings	Leg Curls and Stiff-Legged Deadlifts	2	6, ?, ?	Since hamstrings respond better to low reps, aim for 6 on the first set. You can do a static hold on the last rep of each rest-pause set. This will help maximize tension on the hamstrings.
Traps	Dumbell Shrugs or Dumbell Farmers Walk	1	10, ?, ?	Just do one rest-pause set with the heaviest dumbells you have access to or can handle for 10 reps. Dumbells are shorter in terms of set-up time. Look up at about a 45 degree angle and keep your chest puffed out and shoulders back. This will help activate the traps. To do a Farmer's Walk, you just hold 2 heavy dumbells then walk as far as you can with them.
	Abbreviated Core Combo	4	-	1 set of abs - 1 set of lower back - 2 sets rotator cuff

Cardiovascular Training - None

General Comments:

- Today is Stretch-Pause Training, meaning on your first set, use a weight that you can get 10 reps with. Do the 10, Stretch 20 seconds, then do the OTHER exercise (a stretch-accentuated exercise with a full range of motion), holding the stretch for 3 to 5 seconds on each rep) for as many MORE reps as you can (probably around 4 to 6). Stretch 20 seconds, then finish with as many more reps as you can get on the FIRST exercise again, using only the top, partial range of motion.

- On the stretch exercise, use a weight you could normally get about 12 to 15 reps with.

- As an example, this would look like 10 reps bench press, 6 reps dumbell flyes, 3 reps bench press.

- This layout is the reason for the "?" in the reps column above. Since I don't know how many reps you'll get, I didn't state a rep target - just as many as possible!

- One "set" in this workout means one time through the three mini-sets. THEN take 90 seconds Stretch in between those Stretch-Pause sets.

- If you can, set up your next exercise during the rest period between Stretch-Pause sets. This will help you keep things moving between exercises.

- It's critical that you go for TENSION in the muscles in these sets. Don't just blast out reps. Do them under control and really squeeze the muscles. This will get you best results.

- Write down the weights you use for each exercise so you can track progress and add weight next time you use that exercise again

Muscle Explosion - Workout Sheet - Day 24 - Rest Day.

Bodypart	Exercise	Sets	Reps	Notes
Chest	Flat Dumbell Bench Press and Flyes	3	10, ?, ?	I prefer to use the Swiss Ball for bench presses and flyes. You get better expansion of the chest during the exercise.
Back	Deadlifts	3	10, ?, ?	Use a weight that will really challenge you to get 10 reps. You'll get fewer reps on the next Rest-Pause sets but don't worry about it. Go for broke on the first set. When doing deadlifts, DO NOT do Stretch-Pause training. Because the deadlift is one of THE most effective muscle-building exercises, do a rest-pause set - 10 reps of deadlifts, rest 20 seconds, as many reps of deadlifts, rest 20 seconds, as many as you can get to finish.
Biceps	Reverse Curls and Incline Dumbell Curls	2	10, ?, ?	For the first set, do Incline Curls. On the second set, do Reverse Curls.
Calves	Standing or Seated Calf Raises and Donkey Calf Raises	2	10, ?, ?	Get a good stretch at the bottom of each rep, especially the donkey calf raises.
Traps	Dumbell Shrugs or Dumbell Farmers Walk	1	10, ?, ?	Just do one rest-pause set with the heaviest dumbells you have access to or can handle for 10 reps. Dumbells are shorter in terms of set-up time. Look up at about a 45 degree angle and keep your chest puffed out and shoulders back. This will help activate the traps. To do a Farmer's Walk, you just hold 2 heavy dumbells then walk as far as you can with them.
	Abbreviated Core Combo	4	-	1 set of abs - 1 set of lower back - 2 sets rotator cuff

Cardiovascular Training - None

General Comments:

• Today is Stretch-Pause Training, meaning on your first set, use a weight that you can get 10 reps with. Do the 10, rest 20 seconds, then do the OTHER exercise (a stretch-accentuated exercise, holding the stretch for 3 to 5 seconds on each rep) for as many MORE reps as you can (probably around 4 to 6). Rest 20 seconds, then finish with as many more reps as you can get on the FIRST exercise again, using only the top, partial range of motion.

• On the stretch exercise, use a weight you could normally get about 12 to 15 reps with.

• Remember to hold the stretch position for 3 to 5 seconds on each stretch set!

• This layout is the reason for the "?" in the reps column above. Since I don't know how many reps you'll get, I didn't state a rep target - just as many as possible!

• One "set" in this workout means one time through the three mini-sets. THEN take 90 seconds rest in between those Stretch-Pause sets.

• If you can, set up your next exercise during the rest period between Stretch-Pause sets. This will help you keep things moving between exercises.

• It's critical that you go for TENSION in the muscles in these sets. Don't just blast out reps. Do them under control and really squeeze the muscles. This will get you best results.

• Write down the weights you use for each exercise so you can track progress and add weight next time you use that exercise again.

Bodypart	Exercise	Sets	Reps	Notes
Triceps	Decline Close Grip Presses or Weighted Dips and Tricep Extensions.	2	10, ?, ?	For decline close grip presses, you can use about the same weight for the same reps as you would for flat barbell bench press. We're starting with triceps here as you can use more weight with close-grip presses or dips than you generally can with shoulder presses.
Shoulders	Barbell, Dumbell or Machine Shoulder Press	2	10, ?, ?	Any form of pressing will be fine here. With shoulders, we're not doing any stretch-pause sets, only straight rest-pause training. There aren't any REALLY good stretch-position exercises for the shoulders and you'll get a better mass-building effect with the presses.
Hamstrings	Leg Curls and Stiff-Legged Deadlifts	2	6, ?, ?	Since hamstrings respond better to low reps, aim for 6 on the first set. Be sure to get a good stretch at the bottom of each rep.
Thighs	Squats or Lockout Partial Squats	3	6, ?, ?	Be sure you're getting full squats here to maximize the anabolic effect of the exercise. Do straight Rest- Pause training with the squat. No Stretch-Pause. Squats are one of the best mass-building exercises and we want to take advantage of that here. So do 10 reps, then rest 20 seconds, then as many more squats as you can do, rest 20 seconds, then finish with as many more as you can do.
Traps	Dumbell Shrugs or Dumbell Farmers Walk	1	10, ?, ?	Just do one rest-pause set with the heaviest dumbells you have access to or can handle for 10 reps. Dumbells are shorter in terms of set-up time. Look up at about a 45 degree angle and keep your chest puffed out and shoulders back. This will help activate the traps. To do a Farmer's Walk, you just hold 2 heavy dumbells then walk as far as you can with them. If you do lockout partial squats, skip the trap work - they'll be getting plenty of work supporting the weight.
	Abbreviated Core Combo	4	-	1 set of abs - 1 set of lower back - 2 sets rotator cuff

Cardiovascular Training - None

General Comments:

- Today is Stretch-Pause Training, meaning on your first set, use a weight that you can get 10 reps with. Do the 10, rest 20 seconds, then do the OTHER exercise (a stretch-accentuated exercise, holding the stretch for 3 to 5 seconds on each rep) for as many MORE reps as you can (probably around 4 to 6). Rest 20 seconds, then finish with as many more reps as you can get on the FIRST exercise again, using only the top, partial range of motion.

- On the stretch exercise, use a weight you could normally get about 12 to 15 reps with.

- Remember to hold the stretch position for 3 to 5 seconds on each stretch set!

- This layout is the reason for the "?" in the reps column above. Since I don't know how many reps you'll get, I didn't state a rep target - just as many as possible!

- One "set" in this workout means one time through the three mini-sets. THEN take 90 seconds rest in between those Stretch-Pause sets.

- If you can, set up your next exercise during the rest period between Stretch-Pause sets. This will help you keep things moving between exercises.

- It's critical that you go for TENSION in the muscles in these sets. Don't just blast out reps. Do them under control and really squeeze the muscles. This will get you best results.

- Write down the weights you use for each exercise so you can track progress and add weight next time you use that exercise again.

Muscle Explosion - Workout Sheet – Days 27 & 28 - Rest Days.

INDEX

Pure Physique

HOW TO MAXIMIZE FAT-LOSS- AND MUSCLULAR DEVELOPMENT

Pure Physique is for anyone who ever felt they should be getting more from their efforts in and out of the gym. This book will teach you how to put together an exercise and nutrition program that is truly tailor-fitted to meet your individual needs and goals. Unlike other books that provide fad diets and 'canned' workout routines, Pure Physique was designed with the individual in mind. With this book, you will finally be able obtain the leaner, more muscular body you've always wanted.

Unlike most books in the exercise and nutrition market, this book addresses how to account for differences in needs, goals, abilities, limitations, and preferences.

About the Author

Michael Lipowski is a certified fitness clinician and the President of the International Association of Resistance Trainers. He is a competitive natural Bodybuilder in the INBF, a consultant to other drug-free body builders, and was the personal trainer of the winner of the 2009 Men's Fitness Fit-to-Fat competition. Michael is a writer for Natural Bodybuilding & Fitness and has written for a number of other health and fitness publications worldwide.

Retail Price:	$14.95
Size:	7" x 10"

SPECIAL OFFER

Get this book for 50% off (only $7.48) at **SportsWorkout.com** by using coupon code **MEPURE** during checkout